THE PAIN OF PREMATURE PARENTS

A Psychological Guide for Coping

Michael T. Hynan, Ph.D.
University of Wisconsin-Milwaukee

With Sections by
Lauren Leslie-Hynan, Ph.D.
Marquette University

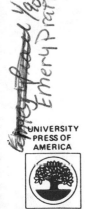

UNIVERSITY
PRESS OF
AMERICA

LANHAM • NEW YORK • LONDON

Copyright © 1987 by

University Press of America,® Inc.

4720 Boston Way
Lanham, MD 20706

3 Henrietta Street
London WC2E 8LU England

Printed in the United States of America

British Cataloging in Publication Information Available

Library of Congress Cataloging in Publication Data

Hynan, Michael T., 1947-
  The pain of premature parents.

  Bibliography: p.
    1. Infants (Premature)—Family relationships.
2. Parent and child.   3. Pain—Psychological
aspects.   4. Adjustment (Psychology)   I. Leslie-Hynan,
Lauren.   II. Title.
RJ250.H96   1987   649'.122   86-28101
ISBN 0-8191-5808-9 (alk. paper)
ISBN 0-8191-5809-7 (pbk. : alk. paper)

All University Press of America books are produced on acid-free
paper which exceeds the minimum standards set by the National
Historical Publication and Records Commission.

Dedicated to:

Joey, Rachel,

all the other unfortunate children, and

their parents

ACKNOWLEDGMENTS

Writing this book has been part of my debt for having a healthy son. For Christopher's life and health I wish to thank the medical staffs of St. Mary's hospital and the Neonatal Intensive Care Unit at County Medical Complex in Milwaukee, WI. I expecially wish to thank Dr. Charles Koh, Dr. John Glaspey, Dr. John Grauz, Dr. Ruth Heimler, and primary care nurses Darla Coleman, Mary Ann Lorenz, and Debby Weishapl.

I also wish to thank numerous other members of the medical staff: Linda Bandoli, Dr. Francine Dvoracek, Dr. Beth Foster, Lillian Guansing, Cindy Hensch, Marilyn Hoffman, Dr. Sally Hunt, Grace Marohl, Dr. Stephen Ragatz, Sister Mary Ruth, Ellen Strutz, Joyce Turner, and Joanne Wetstein. We thank you for your courage, your dedication, and your gentleness in giving Christopher his many enimas and IVs.

In addition, we thank Dr. Donald Cohen for helping to show us that Christopher was a normal baby.

My knowledge of the emotional reactions of parents to prematurity has been aided greatly by the many professionals and premature parents I have talked with and listened to. In this regard I wish to acknowledge Phillip Bagwell, Diane Barnett, Regina Basuel, Susan Blackburn, Jan Finn-Bogason, Dr. Zachariah Boukydis, Dr. Carol Browning, Mary Bures, Susan Burkev, Shari Capra, Bonnie Carpenter, Marcia Corey, Sharon Dalton, JoAnne Fuller, Sandy Garrard, Dr. Peter Gorski, Dr. Page Gould, Dr. Ronald Grocoff, Becky Hatfield, Helen Harrison, Diane Holbrook, Denise House, Chrystyl James, Dr. Thomas Kloor, Debby Lavine, Dr. Henry Mangurten, Dr. Richard Marshall, Lisa Dodd McGee, Dr. Paula Meyer, Lori Meyers, Karen Morrow, Dr. Timothy Murphy, Shari Nance, Linda Orlowski, Terri Palakie, Ed and Martha Paquette, Christine Pelkin, Patricia Piagesi, Dr. Jeffrey Pomerance, Diane Rives, Chris Robin, Dr. Herbert Roffman, Mary Schulte, Terry and Willi Sipes, Richard Smail, Magdi Speros, Barbara Sulek, Patrick Timmons, Barbara Verzo, Leigh Ware, many others whose names I have forgotten, and especially Patricia Hays Evans.

I wish to acknowledge the help of my many typists, copy editors, and proofreaders: Ethel Atinski, Kate Dudley, Julie Gordon, Jim Hynan, Maureen LaWent, Anna Morehouse, Laura Riggle, and Shelly Silfven. I wish to thank Lynn Moen for her suggestions regarding the title of this book. I also wish to express my appreciation to the University of Wisconsin-Milwaukee, Marquette University, and Justus-Liebig University, Giessen, West Germany for their support in writing this book and coping with Christopher's birth.

Lauren and I wish to acknowledge our parents and grandparents (James and Rosemary Hynan, Andrea Leslie Graves, and Josephine Kennedy), our families, and our support network of friends. Without them we would be carrying many more scars of prematurity. Thanks especially to Vince Adesso, Robin Arndt, Rebecca Bardwell, Page and Tim Bristow, Ken and Julie Czisny, Barbara Daniels, Jim Dick, Bob Esch, Julia Hannay, Tom Holcomb, Rev. Michael Ivers, Perry Mueller, Mary Jane Mundt, Vernie Lund, Gary Oltmans, Donna Recht, Erich Schmidt, Tom Sobon, Patty Stevenson, Tom and Mary Taft, Ray and Carol Weiss, Don Williams, and Suzie Williams.

Finally, I would also like to thank James Lyons and the board of directors of University Press of America for recognizing that a self-help book could also be a scholarly book.

TABLE OF CONTENTS

This book was written to help parents adjust to the crises caused by having a premature baby. When my son was born prematurely there were no books on prematurity for parents. As I attempted to understand what was happening to my family, I read through books and journals on obstetrics and neonatology. Later I devoured the books written for premature parents. Scattered in these books were descriptions of the emotional difficulties premature parents face. I was amazed to find that many of those descriptions fit my experiences and those of many premature parents I have talked with.

It is no secret that parents of premature or high-risk infants need emotional support in coping. The emergence of parent groups throughout the USA and international organizations like Parent Care attest to this grass roots movement. This book carries on the tradition of parents helping parents.

I have combined my background as a clinical psychologist with my experience of being a premature parent in writing this book. I describe the common difficulties of prematurity and how these problems affected my family and many others. I also give advice about how you can adjust to your situation.

I hope that both parents and medical professionals can benefit by knowing the sequence of crises in prematurity. Understanding how these crises affect parents is the first step in coping.

INTRODUCTION

Prematurity brings a sequence of predictable crises. Dreams of a healthy new baby are shattered and replaced by fear of death. Mothers go home from the hospital depressed because their babies remain and guilty over a less than perfect childbirth. Families are frustrated and scared by the ups and downs of a baby's recovery. Even when recovery occurs, parents worry about the future development of their baby.

The chapters in this book cover the sequence of these crises, from preparing for prematurity to bringing the baby home. Each of these crises presents a different challenge to parents. For each new crisis there are different emotional reactions which make coping difficult. In each chapter I describe the different crises and give advice about how to adjust. My wife, Lauren, wrote the sections on maternal depression and breast-feeding.

The emotions of prematurity are painful. I wrote this book with the understanding that these painful emotions are also normal reactions to crisis. Many premature parents think they are going crazy because they feel a confusing mixture of panic, depression, guilt, anger, grief, and frustration. Premature parents want to make the pain disappear completely, but this is a losing battle because the feelings are normal--shared by all premature parents.

Accepting the pain and the loss of dreams is very hard. But, once accomplished, parents realize that life again can be good.

CHAPTER ONE

PREPARING FOR PREMATURITY

On July 28th, 1980, my wife, Lauren, had an
emergency operation and gave birth by Caesarean
section to our son. He was eight weeks premature and
weighed two pounds, ten ounces. The experience upset
our lives tremendously. Like other premature parents,
we required a long period of time to adjust physically
and emotionally to the crisis (Kemp & Page, 1986).

Because my wife and I are both psychologists, we
had some advantages during the adjustment. We
benefited from our knowledge of psychological
reactions to extremely stressful situations. Although
we could help ourselves emotionally with this
knowledge, we also found that we needed a great deal
of help from others. The advice and encouragement of
doctors and nurses were very reassuring, but Lauren
and I recognized that they didn't know about our
crisis first-hand. I looked for more personal sources
of support and information.

We were comforted greatly by talking with other
parents of premature infants. In addition, I went on
a furious search for books on prematurity for new
parents. I found almost nothing in libraries and
bookstores, so I thought of writing a book for those
of you who are looking for what I failed to find.

I hope that this book will help you to cope with
the emotional turmoil which accompanies a premature
birth. This book is not intended to be a text of the
medical problems facing high-risk infants or their
parents. You should rely on your physicians and other
books for that information. Instead, I hope to give
you advice and support for the difficulties you will
be facing as you go through the stages of adjusting to
your premature child.

Since our son was born, other books have been
written for parents of premature children. Many of
them are valuable and will help you in different ways.
Born Too Soon: Preterm Birth and Early Development,
by Susan Goldberg and Barbara DiVitto (1980),
describes the patterns of intellectual and emotional
development in premature children. If you are
concerned with the development of your baby during the

1

first year, you will find that the research described in Born Too Soon is very informative. A second book, Premature Babies: A Different Beginning, by two doctors, William Sammons and Jennifer Lewis (1985), is a sensitive and comprehensive description of medical and social difficulties which premature parents must face.

Three other books have been written by parents of premature babies. These books are: Premature Babies: A Handbook for Parents, by Sheri Nance (1982); The Premature Baby Book, by Helen Harrison and Anne Kositsky (1983); and The Littlest Baby, by Fred Pfister and Bernard Griesmer (1983).

I recommend all of these books highly. They cover every detail of the problems faced by premature babies and their parents. They also are written with the perspective that only parents of premature babies can have. My book differs from these five in that I do not emphasize the medical problems facing your baby. Instead, my main focus is to help you, as parents, adjust psychologically to the sequence of crises you will be facing.

Each year, between 250,000 and 300,000 children are born prematurely in the United States. Research shows that prematurity occurs in eight to ten percent of all live births in the U.S. (Usher, 1981; Wertilman, 1981).

An infant is considered to be premature if birth occurs before the end of the thirty-seventh gestational week. (The normal-term infant is born at forty gestational weeks, so a child born two weeks or more before the due date is considered premature.) In addition to the length of pregnancy, another important concern is the birth weight of your child. Children who weigh less than five-and-a-half pounds at birth are considered to be low birth-weight children.

Both the degree of prematurity and the birth weight are important factors in determining the amount of stress you will be experiencing. "Will my baby die?" is a question that can only be answered by giving you the odds of survival for someone as small and as premature as your child.

What most people do not know (and what I didn't know) is that there has been a tremendous improvement in survival rates for premature children in the past few years. I have found books on childbirth written ten or fifteen years ago (and still available in bookstores) which stated that the odds of my son's survival were between ten and fifty percent. However, medical advances and improved technology have dramatically increased the chances that premature babies will grow into healthy children.

For example, children born two to three weeks premature and weighing between four-and-a-half to five-and-a-half pounds now have virtually the same survival rate as normal-term infants (Usher, 1981). Very small babies (like my son was) who are six to eight weeks premature and weigh as little as two-and-a-half pounds have a better than ninety percent survival rate when treated in a neonatal intensive care unit (Usher, 1981). Even the tiniest of babies between one pound, twelve ounces and two pounds, four ounces have a survival rate of approximately seventy percent in a neonatal intensive care center (Cohen et al., 1982; Worthington, Davis, Grausz, & Sobocinski, 1983).

So the odds are very good that your child will live. By the time you read this book, medical advances will probably have made the survival rates even higher. If your doctor tells you that your new tiny baby is doing fine and has an excellent chance for survival, believe it. Your doctor is not saying this just to make you feel better. It's true.

Suspecting Your Baby May Be Premature

Most expectant parents do not anticipate that they will be that one couple in ten or twelve who will have a premature baby. There is an unfortunate tendency to expect that there is always a full nine months to get ready for childbirth. This results in expectant parents who plan to attend childbirth classes in the eighth or ninth month of pregnancy. One of the stresses of a premature birth is that the preparation for childbirth never occurs if it has been put off to the end. It can never hurt you to learn what to do early, and then practice when you have the time later.

There are a number of symptoms which indicate possible difficulties during pregnancy. Examples of these are high blood pressure, excessive swelling of hands and feet, blurred vision, and vaginal bleeding. Your doctor has probably given you a list of these possible complications and told you to call if any occur.

The first sign of Lauren's difficulties was high blood pressure detected during a routine check-up. This was the initial indication that she was developing the medical condition known as toxemia. Toxemia is frequently one cause of prematurity. We were not excessively worried at the time because there were no other physical symptoms to cause alarm. And, we didn't even know what toxemia was.

If you find yourself developing one of these symptoms, or suspecting that you might have a problem, please do two things. First, go to see your doctor. If what is happening is a real problem, it will not go away if you ignore it. If it is not a problem, your doctor will be able to tell you not to worry about it. Second, follow your doctor's advice.

In hindsight, Lauren and I could have done a better job of following our doctor's orders to get a lot of rest after his discovery of her rising blood pressure. Because we are university professors, we were concerned with preparing for classes and doing research, and we were reluctant to reorganize our time.

If there is any concern about prematurity, your task at hand is to buy time for your baby. During the later stages of pregnancy, a fetus develops and grows about an ounce a day. A week or two of additional time may be crucial. Your doctor's advice and treatment are directed at helping your baby develop as much as possible.

If you suspect or know that your baby may be premature, you are certain to become upset. If you are ordered to rest, the anxieties you feel may make complete relaxation quite difficult. Indeed, after talking with many premature parents, I believe that the anxieties about prematurity and the pressures of everyday life make complete relaxation impossible. You must try to accept that you will always be feeling some anxiety and nervousness during this time. If you can accept this normal reaction, you will avoid the danger of emotional over-reaction.

Over-reactions occur when people panic because they are having difficulty controlling or forgetting the initial anxiety. By realizing that some nervousness is normal, you can cope with it and achieve enough relaxation to help your baby. Don't aim for total relaxation--it's a goal you can't achieve. Trying to achieve it will frustrate you and produce over-reaction. It is much better for you to learn to live with the normal anxieties of your situation.

Use whatever coping skills have been successful for you in the past. Some people find meditation or relaxation training helpful. Whatever works is right. This may require that you hire a babysitter to care for your children while you rest, but don't be reluctant to do it. It is important for both you and your baby.

Another difficulty which arises during this time is that you are probably very sensitive to subtle sensations in your body. Any unusual feeling may make you think, "Is the baby coming?" A week before our son was born, Lauren woke up during the night with a feeling of cramping in her stomach. It went away and then came back again. Lauren thought to herself, "Oh my God, the baby's coming already."

You may be hesitant to call your doctor if what you feel is not on the list given you. But when in doubt, call. I realize there are many excuses to avoid doing this: the problem seems small, the doctor is very busy, the doctor will think I'm a hypochondriac, etc. However, when something like this occurs, it disturbs your relaxation and peace of mind. This, in itself, is a good reason to call the doctor. The advice you receive will generally serve to calm your fears, and that alone makes the call worthwhile.

We did not call our doctor that night because Lauren's pains disappeared after she got out of bed and defecated. She assumed that they were just gas pains (they probably were contractions) and went back to sleep. However, if the pains had continued, we would have notified the doctor.

Knowing that Your Child Will Be Born Prematurely

Sooner or later, the time comes when high-risk

parents <u>know</u> that there are difficulties with the pregnancy. Some expectant parents know that a pregnancy will be high-risk even before they conceive. Those parents can benefit from a recent book about sustaining a high-risk pregnancy (Robertson & Berlin, 1986). Most, however, do not anticipate difficulties. When problems occur, parents often find coping difficult.

Three days after Lauren had the "gas pains," she called out to me from the bathroom about 3:00 a.m. I awoke with the same feeling of panic that had wakened Lauren a few moments earlier. When I got to her, she was sitting in the bathtub alongside a large clot of blood. Bleeding was on the list of serious problems, so I called our doctor--at that point, not very concerned about waking him. He instructed us to come to the hospital.

The initial shock of a situation like this usually results in emotional upset and disorganized attempts at coping. Luckily, after the initial shock, most people are able to respond adequately. Hans Selye (1956) has described three stages of reaction to stress called the General Adaptation Syndrome. What Lauren and I felt that night was the first stage, the Alarm Stage.

In the Alarm Stage, people react to the initial shock and then cope with the danger they see. In the second stage, called the Resistance Stage, people adjust to the crisis with maximum levels of adaptation. If people deplete their emotional and physical resources during the Resistance Stage, they experience the last stage, the Exhaustion Stage. In the Exhaustion Stage, people are not capable of adaptive functioning. My purpose in writing this book is to help parents effectively cope during the Alarm and Resistance Stages. If you do this successfully, you can avoid the Exhaustion Stage.

Entering the Alarm Stage is normal, even though the physical and psychological reactions are unpleasant. You will find yourself becoming tense and nervous, you will be concerned only with controlling your crisis, and you will also forget things and make mistakes.

As Lauren and I look back on that night, we are amazed at how well we coped. Somehow, in the face of enormous fear, we managed to dress, pack a few essentials, put the blood clot in a jar, and drive twenty miles. During the drive I needed all my concentration just to see through my tears and keep the car on the road.

The odds are very good that most of you reading this book either have experienced or will experience the Alarm Stage during your pregnancy. Knowing that alarm is a normal reaction to stress should help you in coping. It also helps to recognize that your attention will often be narrowed and focused only on the problems at hand. Because of this, you will miss or ignore other things. Sometimes this can lead to a state of confusion because what you ignore may be important.

For example, when I talked to our doctor he instructed me to bring Lauren to the Labor and Delivery Section of the hospital. All I remembered when I was driving to the hospital was "Delivery," and I drove around the hospital looking for a "Delivery" sign. I am thankful that there was no such sign, or I would have brought Lauren to an empty loading dock. Lauren was aware enough of my confusion to tell me to drive to the Emergency entrance where we were taken care of.

It can be beneficial during the Alarm Stage to realize that confusion will be a part of your adjustment. Realizing this, there will be a smaller chance of becoming upset over silly mistakes (like I made). Accepting confusion will help you refocus your attention on the major task at hand.

Being Hospitalized

No one is emotionally prepared for an emergency hospitalization. Even those of you who are prepared for a high-risk pregnancy (or are facing your second high-risk birth) realize that being hospitalized is upsetting. There will be a great deal of activity upon your arrival. If you have been admitted on an emergency basis, the hospital staff may take action first and explain what they are doing later.

When Lauren was admitted, she was immediately attached to a fetal monitor. The monitor recorded both the baby's heart rate and Lauren's contractions. Lauren was also put on intravenous (IV) feeding. This was done rapidly with brief explanations.

We were told that the major concern of the doctors was the possibility of a premature separation of the placenta from the uterine wall (this can cause bleeding and the onset of labor). We realized that Lauren was being prepared for an emergency Caesarean section. Also, we were told that the fetal monitor indicated that our baby's heart beat was strong and steady. Our fears lessened somewhat, but if we had been given more information (or asked for it), we would have rested even easier.

A good example of the importance of information is our experience with the fetal monitor. Lauren and I watched the fetal monitor throughout the night in case anything went wrong. The steady heart rate was reassuring, but every so often the heart rate went down to zero, stayed at zero, and then came back to normal. You can imagine the panic we felt. It wasn't until we notified the nurse and asked questions that our fears subsided.

It is very normal to observe that readings on the monitor change quite a bit even though the baby is doing fine. Whenever the infant moves inside the uterus, the reading may change and become inaccurate until the electrode attachment to the stomach is moved to where it picks up the heart rate again.

The point I wish to make with this example is the importance of asking questions whenever you have them. No question is too trivial to ask if it concerns you. The answers to your questions can often help you cope, and anything that helps you adjust to the situation will help your baby.

Lauren and I held hands throughout that night and both of us tried to rest. We felt very sad as we heard the sounds of a perfect full-term baby being born in the adjoining room.

The doctor scheduled a number of medical tests for Lauren the next morning. The results of these tests gave us some needed relief. An ultrasound exam indicated that the placenta was correctly positioned and that our baby had good movement. Lauren continued to bleed only slightly and the contractions seemed to have stopped. However, Lauren's blood pressure was still high and the ultrasound suggested that our baby

was small for gestational age. There was still ample
cause for concern. Because Lauren appeared to be
stabilizing, she was taken off the IV and moved into
another room.

Stabilization

At this stage in high-risk pregnancies, one of
two things occurs: your condition stabilizes (either
by itself or through medication), or the child is
born. In this section, I'll describe some of the
problems that face parents when the condition
stabilizes. Even though there is some relief in the
knowledge that it's unlikely that your baby will be
born in the next hour, this time is still difficult.

One difficulty with stabilization is the
continuous monitoring. Lauren's blood pressure was
taken every two hours. She grew tired of being
repeatedly asked if she had headaches or blurred
vision. Constant attention was medically necessary,
but it interfered with her rest.

In order to have a better chance at resting,
Lauren was moved to a room away from the maternity
wing. If your room is in the maternity section, get
it moved if at all possible. Most high-risk parents
become depressed by the sight of full-term expectant
couples strolling hand-in-hand; the sights and sounds
of newborns and the joyful noises heard during
maternity visiting hours can be upsetting.

During the stabilization time, husbands can serve
an important function as a buffer against the outside
world. Some people (for example, employers and your
family) will have to be notified that your wife is in
the hospital. Soon more friends and relatives will
find out, and they will want to call or visit. I urge
husbands to do everything possible to keep people from
calling or visiting if your wife has been ordered to
rest. Make sure that she sees and talks only to those
people she needs. Whenever you inform anyone of the
hospitalization, also tell them not to call or visit
unless asked. Place a "No Visitors" sign on the door
of the room (which should be a private one).

Each time someone called or visited Lauren, she
felt obligated to explain what had happened. She then
became upset, and her blood pressure rose even higher.

The wisdom in keeping all unnecessary people away is especially true if your wife is taking medication to inhibit premature labor. In some cases, women are given drugs such as Ritodrine or alcohol intravenously to postpone labor. This may produce side effects (such as becoming drunk or nauseous) which may grow into greater problems with visitors who don't understand the situation.

One way to keep unwanted visitors away is to establish a communications network. Husbands can contact one or two friends and ask them to be information sources. You can then tell anyone who is concerned to call the sources who will be getting regular updates from you.

I should warn you that this won't work perfectly. As more people find out about your hospitalization, the chances of an unwanted visit multiply. Nervous Uncle Fred or Cousin Minnie will be so concerned that they will try to call or visit against your wishes. If they do intrude, politely ask them to leave or tell them that you will call them back later.

Unwanted visitors sometimes come because they need to reduce their own anxieties about you. They don't realize they may cause additional problems. Your job is to be concerned with reducing your own anxieties, not Uncle Fred's. If you are firm the first time, others will hear of it and leave your wife in peace. If you are not firm, others may think it's all right to sneak in for a few minutes, making it difficult to get the rest prescribed. Protecting your wife this way may upset unwanted visitors, but it is important to put your wife's needs first. Remember that as stabilization grows longer, the baby gets larger and stronger.

During stabilization some husbands may have the option of staying with their wives continuously, night and day. If you want to, and if your wife wishes you to stay, go right ahead if hospital policy permits. You may want to arrange time off from work and provide for child care if you have other children. However, husbands should not feel obligated to stay night and day if there is no apparent need. You need to take care of yourself in addition to taking care of your wife.

I went home at night because I needed some relief
from the pressures of the hospital. Although my sleep
was quite disturbed, it was easier to sleep at home
than in a hospital chair. If you go home, make sure
to leave your home phone number at the nursing station
so that you can be contacted. Another benefit in
going home is that your friends and relatives will
become accustomed to calling your home rather than the
hospital. Also, if you have other children, they will
be anxious to see you and find out how Mommy is.

Fathers may also face the question of whether to
have their children visit the hospital. The answer
will depend on how well your wife is doing and the
needs of your wife and children. In many instances,
the answer will be obvious. If you are in doubt, you
should be aware that some children become very upset
when they see their mothers in a hospital and then
must leave them to go home. Hospitals are scary
places for some children, although the unknown may
prove even more frightening. So your children may
need the reassurance of seeing your wife to calm their
fears.

Your children will also adjust better if you can
provide them with an atmosphere of support and
reassurance. If you are fortunate enough to have
relatives or friends living close by, ask them to stay
in your home with your children (even if you are
home). This will help the children to have a sense of
stability during your trips to and from the hospital.

Fathers who are unable to have someone stay in
the home may find it necessary to have their children
live with friends or relatives temporarily. If this
is the case, you need to be aware of the importance of
visiting your children often. Your children will have
anxieties and fears that need to be alleviated by your
personal reassurances and the messages you bring from
Mommy.

During stabilization, it is likely you will go
into the second stage of Selye's (1956) General
Adaptation Syndrome. That is, you may go from the
Alarm Stage to the Resistance Stage. During the
Resistance Stage, which may be quite long, you will be
functioning at your maximum levels of biological and
psychological adaptation to the stress of a difficult
pregnancy. You will find that, as stabilization gets

11

longer, adjustments get easier. This happens for two reasons. One, the stress lessens as your baby gets larger and you come closer to full term. Second, you will find that you become accustomed to coping with stress and that, in itself, makes life easier.

However, there are some dangers during the Resistance Stage. You need to be careful that you don't deplete all your resources. If you do, you will find yourself in the third stage, Exhaustion, where you will be unable to function adaptively.

There are ways to avoid the Exhaustion Stage. It helps to realize that you can't make it through this crisis totally on your own. Rely on the hospital staff for medical support and on your closest friends and relatives for emotional support. The husband is usually the most important source of support for his wife. But for the husband to be of maximum support, he needs to be supported emotionally by others. Because of the male ego, it is difficult for many men to ask for help. Nevertheless, since doing everything oneself is the easiest way to get to the Exhaustion Stage, asking is crucial. You will find that others are very willing to assist.

During the Resistance Stage, your resistance to the stress of the pregnancy will be up, but your resistance to extraneous stresses will be down. For example, you may fly off the handle if your children can't get along or if a nurse appears unsympathetic. Or, should the family pet pee on the carpet, it may feel as though the straw that broke the camel's back has dropped upon yours like a telephone pole. Recognize that this feeling is a normal, unfortunate part of coping. Don't spend all your energy trying to control what you can't control. By accepting the limits of your stress tolerance, you can continue resisting without becoming exhausted.

As periods of stabilization may be short or long-lasting, you can never be sure when your child may be delivered. In those cases where it is best for the pregnancy to be prolonged, your doctor may take measures to stop labor. In other cases, as in maternal diabetes or toxemia, the development of certain symptoms may lead to an emergency delivery which is impossible to prepare for emotionally. Put your trust in the care of the medical team.

We had hoped that Lauren's stabilization would be a long one. During her third day, our doctor told us she could even go home when her blood pressure came down and remained normal. He informed us that the baby would come early, but he couldn't specify how early. We felt there was a week, perhaps two or three weeks, to prepare for the birth, and were relieved.

I left the hospital to go home for the night, finally sleeping well, until I was awakened by a phone call at 6:30 a.m. telling me to come to the hospital immediately. Lauren had taken a turn for the worse, and our doctor had decided it was necessary to deliver our baby as soon as possible.

Chapter One - References

Cohen, R., Stevenson, D., Malachowski, N., Ariagno, R., Kimble, K., Hopper, A., Johnson, J., Uelana, K., & Sunshine, P. (1982). Favorable results of neonatal intensive care for very low birth-weight infants. Pediatrics, 69, 621-625.

Goldberg, S., & DeVitto, B. (1980). Born Too Soon: Preterm Birth and Early Development. San Francisco: W. H. Freeman and Company.

Harrison, H., & Kositsky, A. (1983). The Premature Baby Book. New York: St. Martin's Press.

Kemp, V. & Page, C. (1986). The psychosocial impact of a high-risk pregnancy on the family. Journal of Obstetric, Gynecologic, and Neonatal Nursing, 15, 232-236.

Nance, S. (1982). Premature Babies: A Handbook for Parents. New York: Arbor House.

Pfister, E., & Griesemer, B. (1983). The Littlest Baby Book: A Handbook for Parents of Premature Children. Englewood Cliffs, NJ: Prentice-Hall.

Robertson, P., & Berlin, P. (1986). The Premature Labor Handbook: Successfully Sustaining Your High-Risk Pregnancy. New York: Doubleday.

Sammons, W., & Lewis, J. (1985). Premature Babies: A Different Beginning. St. Louis: The C. V. Mosby Company.

Selye, H. (1956). The Stress of Life. New York: McGraw-Hill.

Usher, R. (1981). The special problems of the premature infant. In G. Avery (Ed.), Neonatology: Pathophysiology and Management of the Newborn (pp. 230-261). Philadelphia: J. B. Lippincott.

Wertilman, M. (1981). Medical constraints to optimal psychological development. In S. Freidman and M. Sigman (Eds.), Preterm Birth and Psychological Development (pp. 17-40). New York: Academic Press.

14

Worthington, D., Davis, L., Grausz, J., & Sobocinski, K. (1983). Factors influencing survival and morbidity with very low birth weight deliveries. <u>Obstetrics and Gynecology</u>, <u>62</u>, 550-555.

CHAPTER TWO

THE TRAUMA OF PREMATURE BIRTH

That night, Lauren's toxemia had gotten worse.
Her blood pressure had risen even more and could not
be controlled by medication. Her legs had begun to
shake and our baby's heart rate had dropped.
Obviously, the pregnancy had become life-threatening
to both Lauren and the baby. Because giving birth is
the only cure for toxemia, the doctor had decided to
do an emergency Caesarean section.

I arrived at the hospital to find Lauren fully
prepared for surgery. The shock of the situation was
so great that I have forgotten some of the details of
what happened. I do remember Lauren was very
frightened. She was receiving oxygen, and she was
vomiting from some medication. I could do nothing
more than hold her hand, talk to her, and stay out of
the way of the doctors and nurses. We felt helpless,
but I realize now that we were helping each other face
the fear. At this stage, this is all you can do for
each other.

Under the best circumstances, I had hoped to be
present at the birth, but I was emotionally unprepared
for watching Lauren being cut open. Even so, I
probably would have gone into surgery with her if our
doctor had allowed it. But he wouldn't let me make
the valiant gesture. He knew that he needed to work
quickly, and he didn't want my hysteria complicating
things. I did not object.

Although I think there are appropriate times to
question the decisions of doctors and nurses and go
against their advice, an emergency like this is
usually not one of them. I urge you to do everything
requested of you at this time. The circumstances
force you to put all your trust in the medical staff's
knowledge and skills. They have learned to think
clearly during emergencies and adjust to the stresses
of a high-risk birth (Marshall, Kasman, & Cape, 1982).
On the other hand, your own thoughts are likely to be
very muddled and confused by fear. You should ask
them questions to clarify what is happening and what
will be done. Their answers, being the best possible
answers, will reassure you.

After watching Lauren being wheeled from her room
into surgery, I prayed, called my family, and tried to
keep myself emotionally together. I knew this was the
best I could do. Lauren would soon be unconscious
from general anesthesia; I couldn't comfort her. I
tried to be ready to accept the worst should it occur,
although I had a firm belief that the baby would be
born alive and that Lauren would survive. As you cope
with your waiting, the nursing staff will be more than
happy to provide what you need. If you want company,
just ask for it; if you need privacy, the staff will
find it for you.

The First Sight of Your Baby

I sat alone in Lauren's room, trying not to
tremble. I didn't know how long Caesarean surgery
lasted, but I expected it would be an hour or so. How
wrong I was! I had probably been waiting only fifteen
minutes when a pediatrician walked into the room. I
stood up and, as he shook my hand, he told me I had a
fine son. I almost fell down. He quickly explained
that our boy was very small but that he was doing
well. Taking me by the arm, because I could barely
walk, we went to the nursery.

It is impossible to prepare yourself completely
for the sight of your tiny baby. Your first look will
leave you weak and stunned. It is likely your baby
will be inside an isolation chamber called an
isolette. Beside being very short, your baby may also
be very thin, especially in the arms and legs. Like
me, you will be overwhelmed. For most parents, the
world becomes unreal.

During this time, as before, you should not
expect too much of yoursef. You won't be coping very
well, you will find it hard to think, you will be
emotionally confused, and at times you will feel like
a clumsy child. This is because, when birth occurs,
you are thrust back into the Alarm Stage (Selye,
1956). Your confusion and disorientation are normal.
The hospital staff expects you to feel and act this
way, and they are prepared to help.

Remember your attention is focused on adjusting
to the birth. You will ignore many other things and
probably make some mistakes. I certainly did.

18

Our hospital, like most modern facilities,
encourages early contact between parents and premature
infants (Klaus & Kennell, 1976). The pediatrician
told me I could scrub up and go into the nursery to
touch our son through the portholes of his isolette.
Leading me into the washing area, he held up a scrub
gown for me to put on. Instead of putting my arms
forward into the sleeves, I turned around as though I
were trying on a sport coat and the doctor were a
tailor. Gently chuckling, he showed me the correct
way to put on the gown. Then, opening a scrub pad, he
showed me how to lather it up and instructed me to
wash. He left as I practically scrubbed the skin off
my hands for five minutes.

Somehow, I had the idea that I was supposed to
leave the soap on my hands while touching the baby. I
walked out of the scrub room with my hands covered
with orange, syrupy lather. Our pediatrician was
talking with a group of doctors, and they all broke
into smiles when they saw me. Gently, our doctor led
me back into the scrub room and told me I could rinse
and dry my hands.

I mention my blunders because it is likely you
will make some too. You may be as disorganized as I
was, and you may need things explained to you much as
a child needs step-by-step instructions. Don't worry
about it; this phase will also pass.

After I had finished scrubbing, I was shown how
to open the portholes of the incubator and was told I
could touch my son. I was stunned by how small he
was. Most full-term babies look small but a premature
infant looks minuscule. His feet were only about an
inch long, his head seemed to be the size of a tennis
ball. He measured fifteen, extremely skinny inches
from head to foot.

Like most parents in this situation, I was afraid
I would hurt him so I touched and stroked very, very
gently. I probably looked as though I were touching a
frying pan to see if it were hot. This extreme
caution is quite normal at first, and I only touched
my son once or twice before I took my hands out and
closed the portholes.

A nurse who was watching knew the importance of
early contact and encouraged me to continue touching
and stroking the child. She explained that touching

19

and talking to the baby would let him know he was loved and cared for. She helped me overcome a fear that is common for all parents of premature children. At first, premature parents are afraid that something terrible might happen by touching their baby. The nurse helped me realize that my son was not so fragile. She gave me enough courage to ask for some water so I could baptize him, "Christopher." I am very thankful for that shot of courage because anointing Christopher is an experience I will remember with beautiful emotions for the rest of my life.

As the weeks go by, you will see skilled doctors and nurses care for premature babies. They hold premature infants firmly, pick them up, and turn them over and around during treatment. You may shudder the first time you see this, but you will eventually realize your baby is not as delicate as you thought. Then you will become more skilled and confident in holding and squeezing him. This will take some time, but the bonding process will progress more rapidly the sooner you overcome your fear.

Being Separated from Your Baby

Most parents of premature children miss the experience of holding their baby just after birth. The pain of this separation is especially difficult for mothers who are in a daze after giving birth. Some mothers wonder if they really had a baby.

The problems of separation are lessened if the baby remains in the same hospital as the mother. As soon as the mother is able to move about or be moved safely, she can go to the nursery to see her baby and begin the bonding process. The separation is much more difficult when the baby must be transported to another hospital.

Often, if the baby is to be taken to another hospital, a transportation team, wheeling a cart of medical equipment and the isolette, will stop by the mother's recovery room before leaving. You mothers may find that this brief look at your baby can be confusing and emotionally painful.

You are probably still under the influence of a pain killer--the world seems unreal. Your head may be spinning, and it is difficult to focus on your baby or even concentrate. It may be painful to turn over or

sit up to look, and chances are you will not see your
child clearly. After a short while, the staff takes
the baby away again. You may not even be able to pay
attention to what happened. And you are probably very
frightened.

Because this is a very painful experience, you
may choose not to see your baby before another
separation. However, many mothers are afraid that the
baby may die and wish to see their baby alive.
Regardless of how you react, this brief look begins
the bonding process for you, helping you to believe
that you did, indeed, give birth to a child.

I was with Lauren when the transport team brought
Christopher into the recovery room. She was just
coming out of general anesthesia, and she was vomiting
while being fed intravenously. She could not attend
to much beside her own pain and fear.

Lauren scarcely remembers first seeing
Christopher. When she looked at the isolette, all she
could say was, "It's hard to believe anything good
could come of this." She was echoing a common feeling
of mothers at this time. But she did realize she had
a baby, and bonding began.

There are benefits from this experience even
though it is very upsetting. The more you can accept
the fact that the terror is beyond your control, the
better you will be able to cope. And you are left
with hope that your baby will live.

In some premature births, the doctors may be
unsure if a baby needs to be transferred to a hospital
with a neonatal intensive care unit. Many hospitals
without such an intensive care unit provide good
medical care for larger and longer-term premature
babies. In most cases, this decision will be obvious.
When it is not, or when parents are consulted by
physicians for input, they may be faced with a
dilemma.

Although your baby's staying in the same hospital
eases the difficulties caused by separation, your
hospital may not be able to provide the necessary care
if the child takes a sudden turn for the worse.
Emotional needs are, thus, balanced against an added
risk.

If you find yourself in this impasse, my advice is simple. Have your baby transferred to a neonatal intensive care center (Cohen et al., 1982; Colen, 1981). (In fact, in those rare instances when you have serious concern about the adequacy of medical treatment, demand a transfer.) The problems of separation can be overcome. Inadequate medical care often cannot.

The Father's Early Role in Bonding

During the first few days after birth, the father plays an important role in providing a link between mother and baby (Parke, 1982). Even though he is often emotionally upset at this time, he is generally better able than the mother to understand what has occurred. Although the mother has the most intense bonding in most normal births, with premature children the father often has more early contact with the baby than the mother.

Fathers can tell their wives about the baby's condition and appearance. If the baby has been transferred, I recommend that fathers travel to see the child as soon as their wives have recovered sufficiently. If the other hospital is too far away (sometimes babies must be transferred hundreds of miles), fathers should call the intensive care nursery an hour or two after the baby has arrived. This will give the medical staff enough time for an examination and they can provide up-to-date information.

During the first few hours (and days), you undoubtedly will have fear and concern about your baby's survival. Routine contact with the nursery can help to calm you. The doctors and nurses will tell you about your baby's condition, explain the treatment he (or she) is receiving, and answer your questions about survival and any medical problems.

During your first visit, however, realize that the doctors have had only a few hours to examine your baby and may be unwilling to say anything definite. You should expect that they will be very truthful with you. In these situations, doctors have learned it is best to be as accurate as possible in giving information. What you are told will be neither overly optimistic nor pessimistic. No doctor will be able to guarantee that everything will be fine. You will have to live with some uncertainty. But you will feel better for having learned what you could.

For example, I was told that Christopher had about a ninety percent chance of surviving. Laboratory reports indicated that his heart and lungs were working well, although his breathing was irregular. I was also told to expect that he would need a variety of medical treatments. It is common for premature babies to need extra oxygen, to be fed intravenously, to receive blood transfusions, and to be placed under blue lights for jaundice. Because I was informed, Lauren and I were less alarmed when Christopher later received these same treatments.

The father's trip to the nursery is also important because your baby is beginning to recognize you. Babies can hear you, see you, and feel your touch. Indeed, research has shown that newborns in nurseries respond more to their mothers' voices than other female voices (DeCasper & Fifer, 1980). When you begin the bonding process, be sure that you touch your babies, talk to them, and tell them who you are. While facilitating bonding, you will also be facilitating their development. Premature infants are handled by many people in the hospital. Even though it may not look like they respond to your words and caresses, they are aware of what is happening.

When fathers come back from the intensive care nursery to see their wives, they should report about the baby in detail. It may be important to tell your wife all the medical information first. But don't neglect to inform her of the baby's appearance--size, eye and hair color, anything and everything your baby did. This will facilitate the bonding process for her and help her to realize more fully that she actually had a baby.

Most intensive care nurseries have Polaroid cameras. If no one else thinks to take a picture of the infant during your first visit, make sure that you do. If they don't have a camera, bring one for your next visit. Some parents even bring a video recorder and record their baby's movements. Portable audio cassette recorders can also help to start the bonding process between mother and baby. When you record the cries, gurgles, and other noises your baby makes, you are allowing your wife to experience her baby in another way.

23

Still, many premature fathers have told me they felt helpless because they had no control over what was happening to their families. It is certainly true that fathers cannot make things right again--one would like to snap one's fingers and magically have a healthy wife and infant. But two things can help you as you face the despair of powerlessness. One is to realize that your feelings are normal and shared by almost every father in your situation. You must simply accept that there are many things beyond your control. Secondly, understand that what you can do as a father is important. At the height of a crisis, these "little" things seem trivial, but over time you will realize that you have helped bring your family closer together.

Feelings of Grief

During the first few days after birth, most new parents experience a common emotional state. Researchers observing parents of premature infants have called this a state of anticipatory grief (Cramer, 1976; Lindemann, 1944; Parkes, 1972). Anticipatory grief is caused by fear that your baby may die, which leads you to feel grief and sorrow. Anticipatory grief is a very unpleasant, but very normal, reaction. The terrible possibility of death is uppermost in your mind, and you try to cope with what might happen by grieving.

Anticipatory grief, like other reactions to crisis, has good and bad aspects. Its benefit is that it somewhat reduces the intensity of suffering you feel. For example, parents of premature children sometimes delay giving their baby a name. They expect that if they named the baby they would become more attached and feel even worse if the baby were to die than if the baby had remained unnamed.

Even though I baptized Christopher, I avoided officially naming him for four days. He was known as Baby Boy Hynan. I avoided telling anyone (other than family and close friends) that Christopher was born. I felt that, if he were to die, it would be easier for me to lie and say that Lauren had miscarried. I would not have to tell people he was born only to live a few hours and die.

Although this reduced my emotional upset a bit, it had the disadvantage of delaying the process of

attachment and bonding. As human beings, it is
natural for us to do many things which reduce intense
suffering, even if these same things also have
negative effects upon us.

I hope that while you are feeling anticipatory
grief you will remember that it is only a stage to
work through and go beyond. It is important to become
attached to your baby even though grief interferes
with attachment. As soon as you feel comfortable with
a name, give it to your baby. Even though you might
initially feel worse should the child later die, the
long-term emotional recovery of parents from an
infant's death is more rapid if they have named the
baby (Lindemann, 1944).

Coping with a Handicapped Premature Baby

Although all parents of premature babies fear for
their infant's death, many of us have the hope that,
if we are lucky, our children will grow up normally.
If your infant has a physical abnormality, you may be
deprived of this hope. Certainly, your turmoil is
much more intense than that of parents who have
"lucky" premature births.

A handicapped baby presents a doubled crisis.
Your life during the first weeks will seem like a
shattering nightmare from which you may never recover.
I believe that psychological adjustment to this
situation is more difficult than to an actual death.
However, many, many parents have emotionally recovered
from having a disabled baby to find that their lives
can be just as full, if not fuller, of love and joy as
those of parents of nonhandicapped children.

Doctors who have cared for congenitally malformed
babies have described a sequence of stages of
adjustment for parents (Drotar, Baskiewicz, Irving,
Kennell, & Klaus, 1975; Irving, Kennell, & Klaus,
1976). The first reaction is one of overwhelming
shock, accompanied by feelings of helplessness and
sorrow. Next comes denying or minimizing of the
handicap. After this stage of disbelief, parents
generally accept the disability, expressing sadness
and anger. Sadness and anger gradually decrease over
the following months until equilibrium has been
reached, at which time parents discover they are
becoming comfortable with the situation. This comfort
is accompanied by feelings of confidence in their

ability to care for their baby. The last stage is one of reorganization. Parents find they are enjoying caretaking, have formed a positive, long-term attachment to their child, and have adjusted to the crisis.

Please be aware that different parents progress through these stages at different rates and not all parents experience all stages. If your baby is handicapped, I suggest that you read the details of what these experts have written about adjustment to a handicapped child (Drotar et al., 1975; Irving et al. 1976; Korones, 1986; Oehler, 1980).

I also encourage you to read a beautifully written story by Helen Featherstone (1980), a parent of a disabled child. I hope that these direct accounts will help you.

Remember that your adjustment will be slow and may take many months. It is important to know that, although these stages are painful, they are necessary for you to form a positive acceptance of your child's handicap.

It may also help you to talk with other parents of handicapped children. There are support groups which have been organized by parents whose children have some of the more severe disorders associated with prematurity such as spina bifida and intraventricular hemorrhage.

Coping with the Death of Your Baby

By the time you are reading this book, Christopher will be more than six years old. Every once in a while I remember just how fortunate my family has been. I feel very sad when I realize that some of your babies will lose their life-and-death struggles.

If your baby dies, your crisis changes. Instead of fighting for life, you are facing the acceptance of death. There are eloquent articles and books available which can help you through your grief and sorrow (Berezin, 1982; Kennell & Klaus, 1976; Kubler-Ross, 1969). Please read them for emotional support. You will find they describe a process of adjustment similar to that undergone by parents of handicapped children (Arnold & Gemma, 1983; Bordow, 1982).

You may be offered the opportunity to see and hold your baby as a final farewell. This may occur during the last living moments or shortly after your baby's death. Although you should not feel obligated to see your infant if you know that you are emotionally unable to do so, many parents have found that holding and kissing their babies good-bye was an important, valuable experience for them. It can be very helpful in beginning to resolve your grief. If you want to hold your infant one last time, I recommend you do; be aware that it will break your heart.

You may also face the decision of whether to have a memorial service. Most medical personnel who write about this decision suggest that it is desirable to have some form of service (Kennell & Klaus, 1976; Korones, 1986; Marshall & Cape, 1982; Oehler, 1980). This ritual will help facilitate the mourning process.

If you have other children, a memorial service can begin to explain death to them and help them to cope better with the death of their sibling. Books are also available which will help you explain death to your children (Johnson, 1982; Mellonie & Ingpen, 1983; Oehler, unpublished manuscript).

An expert in the field of high-risk infants, Sheldon Korones (1986), has correctly stated, "Mourning...is an exhausting experience that cannot be hurried or denied" (p. 471). The worst of all possible things has happened, and it will take months to recover. This requires patience and a willingness to accept a painful reality. Often, local hospitals or communities will have parent groups for those whose babies have died. These groups can help by giving support needed to cope and begin living the rest of your lives.

Facing the Future

After his transfer, Christopher was hospitalized about ten miles from Lauren. I saw him the afternoon following his birth and returned to Lauren that night. She was still very woozy from the shock of surgery. The two pictures I brought back showed only his tiny head. As I watched her look at them, I could see she was having difficulty believing that this was really her baby. I described Christopher as best I could so she could get a mental picture of him lying in his

isolette in the nursery. Then we both sat back in our
exhaustion. As we did this, we began the next
difficult phase for premature parents--counting the
days that your baby lives.

Chapter Two - References

Arnold, J., & Gemma, P. (1983). A Child Dies: A
   Portrait of Family Grief. Rockville, MD: Azcen
   Systems.

Berezin, N. (1982). After a Loss in Pregnancy: Help
   for Families Affected by Miscarriage, a
   Stillbirth, or the Loss of a Newborn. New York:
   Fireside Books.

Bordow, J. (1982). The Ultimate Loss: Coping with
   the Death of a Child. New York: Beaufort Books.

Cohen, R., Stevenson, D., Malachowski, N., Ariagno,
   R., Kimble, K., Hopper, A., Johnson, J., Uelana,
   K., & Sunshine, P. (1982). Favorable results of
   neonatal intensive care for very low birth weight
   infants. Pediatrics, 69, 621-625.

Colen B. (1981). Born at Risk. New York: St.
   Martin's Press.

Cramer, B. (1976). A mother's reactions to the birth
   of a premature baby. In M. Klaus and J. Kennell
   (Eds.), Maternal-Infant Bonding (pp. 156-166).
   St. Louis: The C. V. Mosby Company.

DeCasper, A., & Fifer, W. (1980). Of human bondage:
   Newborns prefer their mothers' voices. Science,
   208, 1174-1176.

Drotar, D., Baskiewicz,A., Irvin, N., Kennell, J., &
   Klaus, M. (1975). The adaptation of parents to
   the birth of an infant with a congenital
   malformation: A hypothetical model. Pediatrics,
   56, 710-717.

Featherstone, H. (1980). A Difference in the Family:
   Living with a Disabled Child. New York: Penguin
   Books.

Irving, N., Kennell, J., & Klaus, M. (1976). Caring
   for parents of an infant with a congenital
   malformation. In M. Klaus and J. Kennell
   (Eds.), Maternal-Infant Bonding (pp. 167-208).
   St. Louis: The C. V. Mosby Company.

Johnson, J. (1982). Where's Jess? Centering
     Corporation, Box 3367, Omaha, Nebraska, 68103-
     0367.

Kennell, J., & Klaus, M. (1976). Caring for parents
     of an infant who dies. In M. Klaus and J.
     Kennell (Eds.), Maternal-Infant Bonding (pp. 209-
     239). St. Louis: The C. V. Mosby Company.

Klaus, M., & Kennell, J. (1976). Maternal-infant
     bonding. In M. Klaus and J. Kennell (Eds.),
     Maternal-Infant Bonding (pp. 1-15). St. Louis:
     The C. V. Mosby Company.

Korones, S. (1986). High Risk Newborn Infants: The
     Basis for Intensive Nursing Care. St. Louis:
     The C. V. Mosby Company.

Kubler-Ross, E. (1969). On Death and Dying. New
     York: Macmillan Company.

Lindemann, E. (1944). Symptomatology and management
     of acute grief. American Journal of Psychiatry,
     101, 141-148.

Marshall, R., Kasman, C., & Cape, L. (Eds.). (1982).
     Coping with Caring for Sick Newborns.
     Philadelphia: W. B. Saunders.

Marshall, R. & Cape, L. (1982). Coping with neonatal
     death. In R. Marshall, C. Kasman, & L. Cape
     (Eds), Coping with Caring for Sick Newborns
     (pp. 31-46). Philadelphia: W. B. Saunders

Mellonie, B., & Ingpen, R. (1983). Lifetimes: The
     Beautiful Way to Explain Death to Children. New
     York: Bantam Books.

Oehler, J. (1980). Family-Centered Neonatal Nursing
     Care. Philadelphia: J. B. Lippincott.

Oehler, J. (unpublished manuscript). The Frog
     Family's Baby Dies. Available for $1.50 from
     Jerri Oehler, R.N., 210 Landsbury Drive, Durham,
     NC 27707

Parke, R. (1982). The father's role in family
     development. In M. Klaus and M. Robertson
     (Eds.), Birth, Interaction, and Attachment (pp.
     66-74). Johnson & Johnson Baby Products.

Parkes, C. (1972). Bereavement: Studies of Grief in Adult Life. New York: International Universities Press.

Selye, H. (1956). The Stress of Life. New York: McGraw-Hill.

CHAPTER THREE

LIVING THROUGH THE FIRST WEEK

Premature parents face many difficulties during the week after giving birth. The physical and emotional recovery of the mother begins, and there are common problems most mothers face.

If the baby has been transferred to another hospital, mothers are acutely aware that they are alone. Often, the pangs of separation are made worse by seeing others with their new, full-term babies on the maternity unit. Many mothers of premature children prefer not to be reminded of their situation in this way. Most doctors are aware of this and will place them in a room elsewhere in the hospital. If you are put in the maternity wing during your recovery and find it upsetting, just ask to be moved to another unit. Your doctor will be happy to oblige.

A few mothers prefer to recover from birth in the maternity wing. Though they may feel an increase in the sorrow of separation, they find watching other new mothers valuable. They learn about feeding, clothing, and bathing. They may even help the other mothers and thus feel more like mothers themselves while the baby is away.

During this time, you will find that friends and relatives will want to see you. Unfortunately, calls and visits can sometimes interfere with your recovery. Giving birth, especially by Caesarean section, is physically and emotionally exhausting. Peace and quiet will help you recover, but many visitors will disrupt the conditions you need. You may want to review the advice that I gave in the first chapter about this problem and organize an information network to suit your needs. Otherwise, when well-wishers arrive, you will be tempted to relive your hospitalization and, although a certain amount of this can be therapeutic, too much will leave you drained. Your main task is to recover enough to begin relating to your baby. To do this, you must prepare yourself for visiting the neonatal intensive care unit.

Preparing to Visit the Intensive Care Nursery

Before you make your first visit to see your

infant, I suggest you get information that will prepare you for what you will find. What you see will be disturbing (Cohen, 1982). We all picture the ideal baby much as those chubby, happy children seen on television commercials. But your baby will look very different from the Gerber Baby. The difference between this ideal and reality can be shocking.

Often, intensive care nurseries will have some pamphlets which describe the unit and provide pictures of premature infants. You may have been given information like this after the birth. As mentioned in the last chapter, fathers can play an important role in preparing mothers for their first visit to the nursery (Kennell & Klaus, 1982). Fathers who have made previous visits should explain the structure and procedure of the unit in detail, as well as describe the child's appearance. Having some expectation for the first visit will make it seem less overwhelming, although it will remain emotionally intense and frightening.

For example, I explained to Lauren that, of the four sections in the intensive care unit, Christopher was in the critical section. I described to her the procedures for scrubbing up and putting on a hospital gown. Finally, I told her that Christopher had a needle in one of his feet for intravenous feeding, his leg in a sling to protect the IV when he moved, a clear plastic tube going down his mouth into his stomach to relieve gas, and two electrodes taped to his chest to monitor his heartrate and respiration.

However, Lauren didn't expect to see our son until after her discharge. When our doctor suggested we both visit our baby on her fifth day of recovery, it was totally unexpected. She was both excited and afraid as I called the nursery to tell Christopher's primary care nurse that we were coming.

Although, upon arrival, Lauren was quite scared of what she would actually find, her desire to see her baby easily overcame her fear. We scrubbed up and walked hand-in-hand to the nursery. When we came to Christopher's isolette, Lauren took her first good look at him and did what many mothers have done--broke down and cried.

Most intensive care nurseries have chairs handy. If you find yourselves overcome, sit down next to your

baby and let your emotions out. There is no need for
embarrassment; the nursery staff has seen many other
parents break down, and they know it is normal and
psychologically healthy for you to do so.

What you feel is a combination of shock, love,
fear, wonder, anxiety, thankfulness, terror, and many
other emotions. This combination of feelings may be
as disturbing to you as it is difficult to understand.
The best thing you can do is let yourself experience
this volcano. After a while, you will find that the
intensity of your emotions will subside and become
controllable. Then you will be able to begin talking
to and touching your baby.

The nurse will show mothers the isolette, explain
the care the baby is receiving, and will teach safe
ways to handle the child (Harrison & Kositsky, 1983;
Klaus & Kennell, 1983). There is a lot to learn about
how to reach through the portholes to touch your baby.
You will likely feel clumsy, and your first
inclination will be to stroke the hands and feet, then
touch the trunk and finally the head. It will help to
watch the doctors and nurses.

When your baby is healthy enough, you may be
permitted to take it out of the isolette and hold it
for short periods. As time goes by, you will learn
how to handle your tiny child skillfully and will
realize that premature infants must be very strong to
tolerate all the treatments they receive.

Your first visit is an overpowering experience.
There is much to learn and you will not be able to
absorb everything. It is a time to begin relating to
your babies and telling them who you are. Be careful
now and subsequently not to become too tired. It is
better to make your visit relatively short than to
become exhausted. Once you have recovered from your
shock and spent some time with your baby, it may be
wise to go. Although leaving may be painful, you need
time to recover from one visit to the next. When you
leave, be sure to tell your baby that you are going
and that you will return.

The Typical Intensive Care Unit

Modern neonatal intensive care units have many
things in common (Colen, 1981; Korones, 1986; Sammons
& Lewis, 1985). Often they permit visits by parents,

35

and sometimes children and grandparents, twenty-four hours a day. Parents are encouraged to call the nursery any time of day or night to get information about their baby.

You will be required to scrub your hands before entering to minimize the chances of infection. Remember, as you are instructed how to use the scrub pads, that you need only scrub as long as you are told, not until your hands are raw.

Most intensive care units have three or four sections, with the babies requiring the most care in the critical area. All babies in this area will be in isolettes and usually are continuously electronically monitored. As these babies grow stronger, they will be moved to an intermediate care area. Just before discharge, your infant may even be moved to a regular nursery. Thus, you can expect that your baby's isolette will be moved several times during hospitalization.

Sometimes you will be told about a move in advance, but at other times the staff may not have the opportunity to inform you. It is very frightening to walk up to your isolette and find that your baby is not there. You immediately fear the worst, but this is only rarely the case. If anything has gone wrong, you will almost always be notified immediately. Most likely your baby is doing well and has been moved for other reasons. (For example, two or three very sick infants may have been admitted, and your baby was moved into the intermediate area to provide space for them.) Knowing your child may be unexpectedly moved can minimize panic when a move occurs.

As you become accustomed to the intensive care unit, you will notice there is a great deal of activity. In the critical section, there may be as many doctors and nurses as there are babies. The amount of activity and the kinds of treatment may seem shocking initially.

You will watch as nurses put small tubes down babies' mouths so that they may be fed formula. (This is called gavage feeding.) They will insert small IV needles into the babies' tiny veins. Some infants will be under blue bilirubin lights for treatment of jaundice. Others may have oxygen hoods over their heads or endotracheal tubes attached to help them

36

breathe with a ventilator.

In addition, you will occasionally hear one of the electronic monitors sound an alarm. But when an alarm sounds it usually does not mean that a baby is in immediate danger, only that the machine has sensed that the impulses it is receiving have not stayed within the normal range. When this occurs, someone quickly finds the alarm and checks the baby. Sometimes, an alarm sounds simply because the infant has moved, knocking the electrode off and leaving the monitor to receive no impulses. At other times, an alarm may go off merely because a child's breathing has slowed, and a nurse will go over and gently shake the baby to arouse it.

After every visit, you will go through the pangs of separation again. Because a few hospitals have live-in facilities for mothers, you may be able to transfer to where your baby is and keep in close contact. Most of you, however, will be faced with making many trips to see your infant and the difficult emotional task of repeatedly separating.

Waiting out the First Week

Lauren and I reluctantly left Christopher and returned to her hospital. Her blood pressure, which had returned to normal following delivery, had risen again and she needed to be placed on medication. We obviously needed to be careful in how we handled her recovery. Something as beneficial as a visit to Christopher could obviously have unfortunate side-effects.

This is an example of the two-edged sword that is found in quite a few aspects of being premature parents. It took us both a while to recognize that Lauren's physical and emotional recovery was just as important as visits to our son. The recovery process is slow and cannot be sped up without causing additional difficulties. Further, the emotions often take longer than the body to recover. Don't push yourselves too hard. Lauren and I overextended ourselves and suffered for it later.

During the first week of Christopher's life, time went by very slowly. We knew the longer he lived, the better the chances that he would survive. But we continuously feared his death as we counted the

sunrises and sunsets. Every time the phone rang,
every time we walked into the intensive care nursery,
our spines shivered.

All parents finally find themselves facing this
fear and gradually learn to live with it. These
feelings of fear are natural and should not overly
disturb you. As you learn to live with the occasional
panic, and as your baby lives one more day, the fear
will gradually diminish.

When you begin to realize that your baby is
surviving and getting healthier, you stop feeling
anticipatory grief and begin to relate to someone who
will live. But it is not easy to stop anticipatory
grief. You have already taken the risk of deciding to
have a baby, and the worst has almost happened. You
have suffered a great deal, and you have prepared
yourself for your child's death once. It is not easy
to take another risk by expecting your baby to live.

Fortunately, most premature babies survive and
grow up healthy. When you accept this, you will be
more vulnerable to hurt, but you will also feel
greater joy.

When You Have Questions, Ask Them

In your concern for your baby's recovery, you
will have a number of questions. Although you may
feel reluctant to ask them of the busy doctors and
nurses, realize it is important to your emotional
well-being that you do; answers combat fears (Nance,
1982). All doctors and nurses I have talked to
emphasized that they are happy to answer any
questions.

For example, during the first few days of his
life, Christopher didn't gain weight--he lost it. He
went from two pounds-ten ounces to two pounds-seven
ounces. From reading his charts I saw that he was
losing weight. Instead of asking anyone about this, I
just worried. It wasn't until he started to gain
weight that I commented on his weight loss to a nurse.
She told me it was typical for all infants, premature
or not, to lose weight right after birth. I had been
worrying for no good reason. I was upset enough as it
was and didn't need to cause myself additional
anxieties.

Often the staff will try to anticipate your questions and give you as much current information as they can. But even this may seem incomplete or unsatisfying. Get clarification of the details you need.

During a visit, Lauren and I saw that our son was scheduled for another blood transfusion. We had not been informed and were very concerned. We asked a nurse why this was necessary and, as she didn't have the technical knowledge to answer completely, she referred us to a doctor. We wondered about bothering the physician and were reluctant to do so, but she noticed our hesitation and told the doctor our concerns. Our doctor reassured us that the transfusion was a normal part of Christopher's treatment and that Chris was progressing well. If we had not been told, we would have been concerned needlessly.

Asking questions is just one of the ways you have of expressing yourselves during this crisis time. Most parents find themselves in a struggle of trying to hold down their emotions so they can be in rational control. It is best to win this ongoing battle some of the time and lose it some of the time.

It is important for your well-being to let your feelings out periodically. Suppressing them will delay your emotional recovery and the development of your relationship with your child. Hospital staffs recognize that you are in crisis and expect you to be emotional. At times, they may even encourage you to express your feelings instead of holding them back.

Emotional expression is normal and indicates you are adjusting well. Indeed, the staff of an intensive care unit becomes concerned when they see a parent who is always calm, cool, and collected. Outwardly, this calm parent may be handling the situation well, but the complete bottling up of emotions may bring difficulties later.

I am saying that you need to directly express everything you feel. At times you will need to control your feelings to do what you must do. Even to visit your baby, you need to control your fear of finding out that something bad might have happened. Periodically, let yourself loose. Although it may feel like you are losing control, you are in control--

you are permitting emotional expression.

Your Rights as Parents

Many parents wonder what role they have in deciding their baby's medical treatments. At admission you will be asked to sign papers which give consent for your child to have routine care such as blood tests and x-rays. This allows the medical staff to perform the treatments which most premature infants need. When babies are seriously ill, however, parents will be asked to give additional consent for medical procedures which are not routine, such as surgery.

In most instances parents are quite willing to give this informed consent. However, parents should realize that they are entitled to a detailed explanation of the possible benefits and harm that may come from more extensive medical treatments. Parents should also be told of the possible consequences of their baby not having these treatments. This is information which parents have a right to know before giving consent. (This is also true if parents are asked to have their baby participate in research studies of new treatments.)

After receiving these explanations, sometimes parents are not sure that the proposed treatments are best for their child. If this is the case, parents should not feel rushed into making a decision. It is a parent's right to refuse to sign a consent form or to later withdraw consent. It is also a parent's right to get a second or third opinion from other doctors, or to even change doctors. Sometimes getting other opinions will help you feel confident that your baby is getting the correct treatment.

If you find yourselves in this situation please ask the doctors all the questions you can think of. It helps to write down questions as they occur to you and to also write down the doctors' answers. Realize that even with multiple opinions you will not always get an answer about the correct treatment. But it will help you emotionally to know that you have done all that you could.

In some instances parents find that they definitely object to the medical treatments that their baby is receiving. This may occur when parents realize that their baby is very likely to die. Or if

their baby lives, it may be obvious that the baby will
be severely handicapped. At these times parents have
the right to express their feelings that extraordinary
medical procedures be stopped (or not started).

Even though some might feel that stopping
treatment is a selfish decision, many people recognize
that this can be an act full of love for the baby
(Duff, 1981; Lawson, 1986; Stinson & Stinson, 1983).
With blood tests, IVs, intubation, transfusions, etc.,
being a premature baby is painful. Although babies
may not remember the pain, parents are very sensitive
to avoid creating additional suffering when the
outcome of extensive medical treatments is very
pessimistic.

Many times the medical staff will agree that
heroic efforts to prolong a baby's life be stopped.
(Indeed, the doctors may first suggest this to the
parents.) Whether the staff agrees or disagrees with
the parents, this is an emotionally traumatic
situation. If you find yourselves unsure of what to
do, additional opinions may give you direction.

You may be able to consult with an infant ethics
committee. Many hospitals have these committees which
review all the medical information and give advice to
parents. The resolution of this life and death
question never comes easily, but it is always best
when based on open communication between doctors and
the medical staff.

Open communication is the key to the following
"Ten Commandments" which reflect the goals of the best
of neonatal intensive care units (Slade, Reidle, &
Mangurten, 1977):

    I.   Thou shalt talk with parents soon
          after birth.
   II.   Thou shalt be thorough and honest in
          explaining baby's condition.
  III.   Thou shalt be appropriately
          optimistic.
   IV.   Thou shalt avoid difficult medical
          terms.
    V.   Thou shalt encourage parents to see
          and touch baby.
   VI.   Thou shalt share with parents both bad
          and good news about baby.

VII. Thou shalt prepare parents for baby's
death, when it seems inevitable.
VIII. Thou shalt encourage phone calls and
visits.
IX. Thou shalt prepare parents for baby's
discharge.
X. Thou shalt never be "too busy."

At times open communication may be very
difficult, but it is important that you parents try as
hard as doctors do with the above commandments. Your
emotional adjustment depends upon it.

Mother's Hospital Discharge

A mother's trip home from the hospital is often a
time of jumbled emotions. By now you have probably
grown tired of the hospital routine and would like to
return to the comforts of home. However, I advise you
not to rush your hospital stay. Even though your
physical recovery may be sufficient for discharge,
your emotional recovery may take longer.

If you feel very fatigued, or aren't quite ready
to face a home full of children and their demands, it
may be wise to stay in the hospital for an extra day
or two if hospital policy and your insurance will
permit this. No one is going to give you a medal for
a short hospital stay. You need your strength for
repeated visits to your baby.

The comforts of home also bring obligations and
responsibilities--meals to cook, clothes to wash,
cleaning to do, perhaps children to care for. Your
recovery will be facilitated if you make arrangements
to get help with these routine tasks. Although your
concern for the baby will be primary, you may become
discouraged if household chores take too much of your
time and energy.
Doing these chores is another way fathers can be
especially helpful. In most cases, fathers have
already taken on an added burden by doing
housekeeping. Unfortunately, some men expect that,
when their wives return home, the usual division of
labor will be restored.

To help your wife, try to have the home cleaned
before she returns home. Pitch in and do as much

housework as you can for the next few weeks, perhaps asking friends and relatives to help. This will help speed her recovery.

Up until discharge, most fathers have been the primary parent for their premature babies. Fathers often take to this role naturally and enjoy it. However, once the mother returns home, the father's parenting role changes as the mother generally takes a more active role in caring for their infant. Depending upon the family structure, the mother may take equal or primary parenting responsibility. When this occurs, some fathers may experience jealousy which may be upsetting.

I was lucky enough to be aware of my jealousy and realize that it was very important for Lauren to take an active role in caring for Christopher. By giving up my position as primary parent so that Lauren and I could share parenting equally, I gained time which I was able to use doing extra household chores. Although I had reduced the amount of contact I had with Christopher, our contact remained significant. I was his parent too. I did not have to give up any of my joy.

For Grandparents

In the midst of the crisis of prematurity, many people forget that grandparents also have their own worries and emotional reactions (Blackburn & Lowen, 1985). Most grandparents find they have two concerns: They worry about the health of their grandchild and they want to help their child cope with the dangers of being a premature parent.

Many grandparents wish to see the baby during hospitalization but find it difficult to visit the nursery. Sometimes an intensive care unit reminds them of their own failing health and thus makes them reluctant to visit. Although seeing your tiny, sick grandchild will upset you, please visit the intensive care unit if you live within traveling distance. It will help you both to get a more realistic view of your grandchild's treatment and to understand what your child is feeling.

It was difficult for my parents to visit Christopher six days after his birth. They were very shaky when they came to the hospital, and you should expect yourselves to feel the same way. This is quite normal, and you will soon get over your anxieties.

My father's reactions are good examples of how grandparents adapt when they visit the baby. As we were scrubbing up to go into the nursery, he was obviously trembling. I told him it would be all right and led him into the unit. He stood back, uncertain, and watched for about ten minutes until his shock passed. Then he became very involved with Christopher, and soon both my parents had adjusted to the intensive care unit. They were strolling, looking at babies, and chatting about the medical marvels.

Many grandparents also want to protect their children from the anxieties of being premature parents. They remember being worried over the illnesses of their child (or children) and, with good intentions, may tell their child what to do in caring for the baby or other offspring at home. Unfortunately, telling your child what to do or trying to protect him (or her) from bad feelings is not the best way to help now.

Many premature parents have told me there are two things they especially appreciated from their own parents. One is an offer by their parents to do anything needed. This allowed them more control over their own lives. The other is an acknowledgement that what they are doing is very difficult.

You may be asked to babysit for your other grandchildren, assist in breast-feeding, or help with housework. Especially important will be your sharing of how concerned or frightened you were many years ago when your children were sick. If you do this, you will be giving the parents the support they need, and they will appreciate your understanding of them.

The Empty Home

The major source of difficulty when premature mothers are discharged is the obvious fact that most cannot bring their babies home.

When Lauren and I came home, we realized that, even if Christopher made a rapid recovery, it would still be six to seven weeks until he could join us. This, together with our anxieties about his survival,

44

made Lauren's homecoming an uneasy event.

Your house or apartment may feel strange to you.
If you have no other children, your home will
certainly seem empty, especially the room you planned
to turn into the nursery. Millions of premature
parents have had this experience. The feelings of
strangeness are not long-lasting and gradually
disappear.

Let the comforts of home exert their therapeutic
effects as you begin the long wait for the baby's
arrival.

Chapter Three - References

Blackburn, S. & Lowen, L. (1986). Impact of an infant's premature birth on the grandparents and parents. Journal of Obstetric, Gynecologic, and Neonatal Nursing, 15, 173-178.

Cohen, M. (1982). Parents reactions to neonatal intensive care. In R. Marshall, C. Kasman, & L. Cape (Eds.), Coping with Caring for Sick Newborns (pp. 15-30). Philadelphia: W. B. Saunders.

Colen, B. (1981). Born at Risk. New York: St. Martin's Press.

Duff, R. (1981). Counseling families and deciding care of severely defective children: A way of coping with "Medical Viet Nam." Pediatrics, 67, 315-320.

Harrison, H., & Kositsky, A. (1983). The Premature Baby Book. New York: St. Martin's Press.

Kennell, J., & Klaus, M. (1982). Caring for the parents of premature or sick infants. In M. Klaus and J. Kennell (Eds.), Maternal-Infant Bonding (pp. 151-226). St. Louis: The C. V. Mosby Company.

Klaus, M., & Kennell, J. (1983). Adapting to a premature or sick infant. In M. Klaus and J. Kennell (Eds.), Bonding: The Beginnings of Parent-Infant Attachment (pp. 93-119). St. Louis: The C. V. Mosby Company.

Korones, S. (1986). High Risk Newborn Infants: The Basis for Intensive Nursing Care. St. Louis: The C. V. Mosby Company.

Lawson, J. (1986). "Premie - Barbarism"? Parent Care---News Brief, 1, 3-5.

Nance, S. (1982). Premature Babies: A Handbook for Parents. New York: Arbor House.

Sammons, W. & Lewis, J. (1985). Premature Babies: A Different Beginning. St. Louis: The C. V. Mosby Company.

Slade, C., Reidle, C., & Mangurten, H. (1977). Working with parents of high-risk newborns. Journal of Obstetric, Gynecologic, and Neonatal Nursing, 6, 21-26.

Stinson, R., & Stinson, P. (1983). The Long Dying of Baby Andrew. Boston: Little, Brown, & Co.

CHAPTER FOUR

BONDING AND BREAST-FEEDING

In the past chapters, I have written about the importance of bonding. Now I will describe why bonding is so crucial for both parents and their babies. Bonding, the emotional attachments parents develop from contact with their infant, is the basis for love between parents and child. Drs. Marshall Klaus and John Kennell (1983a), well-known experts, believe that this bond forms the basis for all the child's future attachments. The first bonds are established when parents look at, talk to, and touch their baby. However, the bonding process is interrupted in most premature births. Although this brings additional difficulties, they are not insurmountable.

The bonding process begins with conception. When parents decide to create a baby, they form an attachment to their image of that baby. During pregnancy, the woman's body, serving as the baby's temporary home, changes dramatically; she also feels movement. The father begins to form bonds during pregnancy, and these attachments grow stronger after the fetus has begun kicking, especially when the father can see and feel movement on his wife's stomach. Many parents think of, perhaps even call, their unborn child by name. My wife and I called our son "Boomer" because of the way he kicked.

Most parents are continuously aware of the due date, scheduling their lives around it. In full-term births, the gradual bonding process often results in preparedness. But even with a full nine months, many parents are not completely ready to have their child.

It is no wonder that premature parents feel totally unprepared. They suddenly find themselves with a baby they did not expect for another four, ten, or twenty weeks. Despite this, most premature parents adapt beautifully and form deep, loving bonds with their infants.

Bonding for Premature Parents

Prematurity and early separation often give parents feelings of inadequacy. In full-term pregnancies, parents expect to have frequent contact with their new baby. Normally, Drs. Klaus and Kennell (1983b) advocate that mother, father, and infant be alone together thirty to sixty minutes immediately after birth. However, after a premature birth, most parents do not hold their baby for hours or days. Because of this time delay, coupled with their fear of the child's frailty, many premature parents feel awkward initially.

Almost all parents begin to touch their premature babies with great caution, and the barrier of the isolette makes close contact difficult. Some are reluctant even to look at the child at first. But, as bonding develops, parents spend more time talking to their babies, gazing directly into their eyes. This direct eye contact (called the en face position) is a good indication that bonding is developing well.

When babies grows healthier and can be temporarily removed from the isolette, parents learn how to hold them. This touching and holding has positive effects for parents and babies. Over time, babies show improved breathing, greater nervous system development, and more rapid weight gain as a result of being gently held and touched (Klaus & Kennell, 1983c). Drs. Kennell and Klaus (1976) also have reported, "Over many years, we have gained the impression that the earlier a mother comes to the premature unit and touches her baby the more rapid her own physical recovery from the pregnancy and birth process" (p. 120).

Although there are many advantages to early bonding, and the medical staff will encourage you to have early contact with your child, do not allow yourselves to be pushed into bonding too rapidly. There is danger in too much encouragement; you may feel forced to attempt something you are not ready to do. If you are certain you are not ready to do something with your baby, decline the invitation and avoid going through the motions while resisting emotionally. The bonds that you willingly make are the important bonds which, although made gradually, will develop fully and deeply.

Do not be discouraged if you find bonding difficult. With encouragement, Lauren and I changed and bottled Christopher inside the isolette. However, we spilled our share of milk and dropped our share of

diapers into the isolette before overcoming
clumsiness. Remember that the more you try, the more
you will fall in love with your baby.

Problems in Bonding

In some instances, there are parents who are
unable to bond with their premature infant. A mother
or father may avoid seeing the baby for weeks after
birth, if at all. Some are emotionally unable to form
an attachment to a sick baby and do not truly become
parents until the child is well and ready to come
home. In rare cases, premature babies are put up for
adoption because one or both parents refuse to care
for them. This severe disruption in bonding is an
indication of the difficulties all parents of
premature babies experience. Unfortunately, some of
us have greater problems than others.

Often, premature parents fear that there will be
long-lasting harm done to their infants due to
separation after birth. In the past, it was believed
that there was a critical period just after birth
during which bonding must occur if the baby's
emotional and physical growth were not to be stunted.

However, modern research has discovered no long-
term effects upon a child's development which can be
attributed to parental separation after prematurity
(Bradley, 1983; Rutter, 1981). Today, most experts
recognize that, despite the temporary problems posed
by separation, successful bonding occurs eventually in
almost all cases. For example, one study has shown
that, although separation resulted in mothers feeling
inadequate when they began to renew contact with their
babies, almost all of these mothers were able to cope
successfully and become competent parents (Liefer,
Leiderman, Barnett, & Williams, 1972).

The fact that there are millions of well-adjusted
adults who were premature babies is a tribute not only
to modern medicine, but also to the parents who
adapted. Even severe separation may not have long-
term detrimental effects. In some cases in which one
or both parents did not choose to visit their
hospitalized baby, bonding was successful upon
discharge, with the baby developing well in a loving
home.

Some parents feel so guilty about separation that they imagine they are inadequate. If you experience this guilt, express it so that you can be supported by both your family and the medical staff. They can help you to begin bonding at your own pace, and you will discover your natural parenting abilities. As you continue to bond, you will feel more and more adequate as a parent. Your first clumsy touches will become movements that are as assured as they are loving.

The Development of Bonding

Bonding is a continuously changing process, especially during the first few months. Often, the parents' first attachment is to a baby who is very sick. The fear of death may linger long after birth, and it may be hard to realize that the high-risk infant has grown healthy and is thriving.

Parents need to allow their attachments to change as they and the baby develop. If they are not flexible in bonding, they run the risk of relating to the child as someone who will always be sick and frail, acting unnecessarily protective and causing future family discord.

If one parent has realistically bonded to a healthy child, but one still considers the child sickly, the child may receive inconsistent feedback and discipline. One parent may be permissive in child rearing while the other is very cautious. This can make it difficult for the child to develop a consistent self-concept. "Am I healthy, or am I sick?" In order to avoid this problem, parents must be flexible and realistic in how they regard their children.

A well-known expert in baby development, Dr. T. Berry Brazelton (1982), has observed that many parents show predictable changes in how they regard their premature baby. These changes correspond to the development of bonding. According to Dr. Brazelton, most parents initially relate to their baby in chemical and physical terms during the stage just following birth in which they find it hard to believe they have become parents. Their major concerns are such things as the degree of oxygen concentration the child is receiving, blood gases, changes in the baby's pH and weight loss or gain. Many parents memorize the metric weight system because premature babies are weighed in grams, not ounces. (One ounce is equal to 28 grams. This is easier to remember if you think of an ounce as approximately 30 grams.)

As bonding develops, parents change their perceptions and are more concerned with the baby's reflexes than chemistry. Many parents are still detached from their premature baby. The ties between parent and child are still developing, and parents are more likely to comment about the baby's responsiveness to members of the medical staff than to themselves.

Parents begin to consider the baby as theirs when parent-child attachment becomes stronger. They begin to interact more, realizing that their child is a human being who is responding to them as his or her parents; they identify human behavior, such as smiling and turning to listen.

Over time, this bond results in an intimate set of reciprocal interactions between parents and child which has been described as a "dance" by researchers who have observed it (Condon & Sander, 1974). Babies who "dance" move their bodies in synchrony with the voices of their parents, each move timed to respond to the words they hear.

Touching and Handling Premature Babies

Even though I have stressed that handling your baby is important for bonding, be aware that sometimes it is best not to handle babies (Gorski, Hole, Leonard, & Martin, 1983; High & Gorski, 1985). Premature infants have immature nervous systems. Even though they seem to have few responses to what happens around them, research has shown they are very responsive. Indeed, many are easily overstimulated. Their lack of apparent responsiveness protects their nervous systems from becoming overloaded (Als & Brazelton, 1981; Gorski, Davison, & Brazelton,1979; Sammons & Lewis, 1985).

You will find that babies have ways of telling you when they want stimulation and when they have had enough. The best times to interact with babies is when they are alert and have a bright facial appearance. Remember, a very young premature baby is not able to absorb a great deal of handling.

When babies have had enough stimulation, they
will let you know. If they grimace, startle, or turn
away from you, it means they are becoming fatigued.
When babies are overstimulated, they spend extra
calories in grimacing, crying, and turning away.
Overstimulation may result in slow heart beats
(bradycardia) or long intervals between breaths
(apnea). Some doctors also believe that babies learn
to breast-feed better in a very calm, quiet
environment.

When babies are stressed, they arch their backs,
hold their arms up, and extend their fingers apart.
Then it is best to put them down or hold them still so
they can rest. Many babies can be calmed by putting
their arms over their chest so their elbows are close
together. Gently pressing their arms against their
chest also helps (Healey, 1986).

It will take a while to learn how to interpret
your baby's responses. The medical staff can teach
you when it is best to handle your baby and when your
baby has had enough. As babies grow older and their
nervous system develops, they will benefit from
increased interactions with you.

Sometimes premature parents who have heard about
the importance of bonding find it difficult to refrain
from interacting with their baby as much as possible.
This is especially true for those who may only see the
child for an hour every day or two.

If your baby becomes stressed during handling, it
is not a sign of rejection, rather an acknowledgement
that a rest is needed. After the infant has
recovered, another interaction will be welcomed. Take
comfort in the fact that, as your baby grows, it will
want--and demand--much more from you.

The degree of medical care necessary in an
intensive care unit provides a large amount of
stimulation each day (Blackburn & Barnard, 1985).
When you visit, your child may not be alert and ready
to play. Sometimes, your baby may be asleep or
irritable, and it will be hard for you to feel like a
loving parent. Then it is best to let your baby rest
until it gives you that smiling look which invites
your slow and calm interactions.

You can ask your baby's nurse to record those times of day when your baby is most likely to be alert. These times may not be regular each day, but some babies do develop regular cycles of sleep and alertness. If you discover that your baby is likely to be alert at a certain time of day, that is the best time for your visits.

Remember that, if your baby seems indifferent to you, it is not your fault. Your baby needs sleep and rest to grow and develop. Realizing this will give you the patience to wait until your baby is ready to interact with you.

Breast-feeding, by Lauren Leslie-Hynan

Breast-feeding is an excellent way to facilitate bonding between mother and baby. The decision to breast-feed is a very personal one which only you can make.

I had planned to breast-feed my full-term baby, having accepted the findings of researchers that mother's milk provides both good nutrition and antibodies to prevent disease (Gerrard, 1974; Jellifee & Jellifee, 1971). More importantly, I wanted intimacy with my child.

I never reconsidered my original decision after Christopher's premature birth. In fact, I became more adamant about breast-feeding because I was not with him. Providing milk became a strong physical and psychological bond I had with Christopher that no medical staff could provide, assuring me a role in his life.

Although the decision itself was easy, I found carrying it through to be difficult. Because of the degree of Christopher's prematurity, he was not yet able to suck or keep milk in his stomach but had to be fed intravenously, compelling me to "express" my milk.

Expression is the squeezing of milk from the breast. Breasts must be emptied of milk at regular intervals in order to keep milk in good supply. Many doctors advise that expression occur every three to four hours. Milk can be expressed by hand or pump. A trained nurse or doctor can show you the techniques of expression.

Initially, when your baby has developed enough to be nourished by milk, your baby may receive feedings by gavage and, when ready to suck, from a bottle with a special nipple designed to allow premature infants to drink with little effort. I expressed milk for ten days before Christopher was able to take it by gavage; his breast-feeding did not begin until three weeks after birth. Two more weeks had to pass before he began to breast-feed well.

Expression is inefficient compared to a baby's suck. Thus, the total amount expressed will likely be less than the amount available. This often results in the mother providing only a percentage of the baby's milk when the baby is able to begin breast-feeding.

The amount of milk produced is directly related to the amount removed; the more you express, the more milk you'll produce. But, not only does expression take time to learn, once learned it is time-consuming. I expressed twenty minutes every three hours; some mothers express up to an hour at a time.

Success in providing the majority of your baby's milk does not come easily. Given these obstacles, it is not surprising that many women do not breast-feed their premature infants. But, should you decide to, here are some techniques and personal experiences.

Techniques of Expressing

The choice of techniques is one of personal preference and what works best for you.

A common technique utilizes a manual pump. There are many types--cylinder, Lloyd-B, Kaneson, and bicycle horn. All fit around the breast and create suction around the milk ducts in the areola. Manual pumps work satisfactorily for many women and are reasonably priced.

If, however, they do not work for you, you may wish to try an electric pump. Most women find it to be the best and most efficient method of expression. Suction is created by an electric motor that alternately pulls and releases the breast. However, electric pumps are very expensive, and you may prefer to rent one to try it out. You may also wish to investigate whether your insurance company will pay for its use.

Because my areolar area is small, the bicycle
horn pump was not efficient for me. Rather than try
another pump, I decided to learn how to express by
hand. In manual expression, the breast is cupped in
one palm and the thumb is used to push down and across
the milk sacs behind the areola. This action is begun
on one side of and continued around the entire breast
while the other hand holds the container for the milk.
(Plastic nurser bags used as containers can be
immediately sealed with a rubber band and
refrigerated.)

Independent of the method you choose, you may not
supply all your baby's milk. Like me, you may react
by becoming disappointed and overdo expressing. I
initially approached expressing so feverishly that I
pushed and squeezed until my breasts developed
blisters and my fingers felt arthritic!

Many premature mothers try a number of techniques
of expression before they find one that works.
Building and maintaining a milk supply is difficult,
does not happen overnight, and requires a great deal
of patience. If you find that you are producing very
little milk, you are only discovering what thousands
of others have experienced. Keep trying. Even if you
provide only a small amount of milk, your baby will
still be receiving the antibodies and nutrients that
only you can provide.

With any technique of expression, cleanliness is
crucial. Wash your hands and breasts in warm water.
Make certain to clean or sterilize pumps according to
direction. As soon as you have expressed, refrigerate
or freeze the milk in either a sterilized bottle or a
plastic nurser bag.

Whether you refrigerate or freeze milk depends
upon how often you visit your baby. When
refrigerated, milk is only good for twenty-four to
forty-eight hours. Although milk frozen in a
refrigerator freezer can be kept up to two weeks, and
in a deep freezer at zero degrees Fahrenheit for much
longer, thawed milk must be used within twenty-four
hours. Freezing milk also destroys some of its
antibodies.

After my supply developed, I was able to produce
two to three ounces of milk with each expression.
Afterward, I folded down the top of the nurser bag

three or four times, folded the top half vertically, and put a rubber band around it. Before refrigeration, I labeled the bag with Christopher's name, the date, and time of expression.

When Michael and I went to the hospital, we put the nurser bags in a thermos with some ice cubes and, on very hot days, packed the thermos inside a small Styrofoam cooler with more ice. Once at the hospital, we gave the thermos to the nurses, who put the bags of milk in the hospital's refrigerator.

The Baby at Breast: Initial Attempts

Upon entering the nursery one morning, I was told that Christopher's suck had developed enough that he was ready to learn breast-feeding. Although we knew this would be coming soon, it was only five days since he had begun bottle feeding and, although he had been getting milk easily through a "premie nipple," it would be harder to get it directly from my breast. I responded to the news with a "Help!" look on my face. I was thankful when a nurse asked if she could give me guidance.

There are many positions used in breast-feeding, and each mother and child have to find the best one for them. Christopher's first attempts looked more like kissing than sucking. While he did suck a bit, he spent more time cuddling, looking around, and listening. During subsequent days, I tried every position I could think of to get him to feed: I sat down; I stood up; I lay down and put his lips on my nipple; I laid him on his back and hung my breast over his mouth; I cradled him in my arms; and I held him like a football. But for five days nothing worked, even when we arrived in time for his scheduled feeding. I would try to breast-feed for about a half-hour, frustrated to the limit, then express while Michael fed Christopher with a bottle.

But, finally, success came on the sixth day when Christopher grabbed on and sucked! He only took fifteen cc's (one-half ounce), but I was elated. It had all been worthwhile.

However, frustration returned. Progress became very slow and uneven--he would not breast-feed at all for the next seven days, then took forty minutes to consume thirty cc's. But after this, Christopher was

58

able to breast-feed on almost every attempt. Even so, I was never able to provide all his milk during one feeding.

Because the amount of milk consumed is measured by weighing the baby before and after feeding, this measurement is not precise, especially if the infant urinates or defecates. If the weighing shows your baby only to have gained ten grams (one-third ounce), do not be disappointed, particularly if your baby suckled well. Your baby may have lost thirty grams defecating.

Before Christopher was born, my goal was to provide all of his nutrition. After his birth, this goal changed many times. I was naturally disappointed, and a bit guilty, that he needed bottle supplements after almost every feeding, but there was no reason to be. In some cases, the effort involved to breast-feed may be so great that the mother decides, despite all original intentions, not to establish a milk supply. Many successful mothers, both premature and full-term, are not able to breast-feed.

For a few days after our son came home, I tried nursing him every two hours so that supplements would not be necessary, but this proved too exhausting. I could not reach my goal of providing all his milk while maintaining my own recovery.

If you are not the perfect breast-feeder, be easy on yourself; breast-feeding will help bonding only to the extent that your overall recovery continues. As the love between you and your baby grows, bonding will become stronger with each passing day, regardless of your choice of feeding.

Chapter Four - References

Als, H. & Brazelton, T.B. (1981). A new model of assessing the behavioral organization in preterm and full term infants. Journal of the American Academy of Child Psychiatry, 20, 239-263.

Blackburn, S. & Barnard, K. (1985). Analysis of caregiving events relating to preterm infants in the special care unit. In A. Gottfried & J. Gaiter (Eds.), Infant Stress Under Intensive Care: Environmental Neonatology (pp. 113-129). Baltimore: University Park Press.

Bradley, R. (1983). Summary comments. In V. Sasserath (Ed.), Minimizing High-risk Parenting (pp. 25-30). Johnson & Johnson Baby Products Company.

Brazelton, T. B. (1982). Behavioral assessment of the premature infant: Uses in intervention. In M. Klaus and M. Robertson (Eds.), Birth, Interaction, and Attachment (pp. 85-92). Johnson & Johnson Baby Products Company.

Condon, W., & Sander, L. (1974). Neonate movement is synchronized with adult speech: Interactional participation and language acquisition. Science, 183, 99-101.

Gerrard, J. (1974). Breast-feeding: Second thoughts. Pediatrics, 54, 757-764.

Gorski, P., Davison, M., & Brazelton, T. B. (1979). Stages of behavioral organization in the high-risk neonate: Theoretical and clinical considerations. Seminars in Perinatology, 3, 61-72.

Gorski, P., Hole, W., Leonard, C., & Martin, J. (1983). Direct computer recordings of premature infants and nursery care: Distress following two interventions. Pediatrics, 72, 198-202.

Healey, T. (1986). Supporting an Appetite for Life: Treating and Nourishing the Fragile Low Threshold Preterm Infant. Paper presented at the meeting of Parent Care...Making the Difference, Indianapolis.

High, P. & Gorski, P. (1985). Recording environmental influences on infant development in the intensive care nursery: Womb for improvement. In A. Gottfried & J. Gaiter (Eds.), Infant Stress under Intensive Care: Environmental Neonatalogy (pp. 113-129). Baltimore: University Park Press.

Jellifee, D, & Jellifee, E. (1971). The uniqueness of human milk. American Journal of Clinical Nutrition, August.

Kennell, J., & Klaus, M. (1976). Caring for parents of a premature or sick infant. In. M. Klaus and J. Kennell (Eds.), Maternal-Infant Bonding (pp. 99-166). St. Louis: The C. V. Mosby Company.

Klaus, M., & Kennell, J. (1983a). The family during pregnancy. In M. Klaus and J. Kennell (Eds.), Bonding: The Beginnings of Parent-Infant Attachment (pp. 1-14). St. Louis: The C. V. Mosby Company.

Klaus, M., & Kennell, J. (1983b). Labor and birth. In M. Klaus and J. Kennell (Eds.), Bonding: The Beginnnings of Parent-Infant Attachment (pp. 15-34). St. Louis: The C. V. Mosby Company.

Klaus, M., & Kennell, J. (1983c). Adapting to a premature or sick infant. In M. Klaus and J. Kennell (Eds.), Bonding: The Beginnings of Parent-Infant Attachment (pp. 93-119). St. Louis: The C. V. Mosby Company.

Liefer, A., Leiderman, P., Barnett, C., & Williams, J. (1972). Effects of mother-infant separation on maternal attachment behavior. Child Development, 43, 1203-1218.

Rutter, M. (1981). Maternal Deprivation Reassessed (2nd ed.). Middlesex: Penguin Books.

Sammons, W., & Lewis, J. (1985). Premature Babies: A Different Beginning. St. Louis: The C. V. Mosby Company.

CHAPTER FIVE

AWAITING YOUR BABY'S HOMECOMING:

"ALL IT IS, IS HARD"

Each stage of premature parenthood produces new problems. Waiting for your baby to come home is always difficult, even if just for a few days. Waiting for months is an eternity of soul-searching and sadness.

The emotional turmoil of premature birth does not go away quickly; it reverberates. Adjusting to the trauma often takes many months. The human mind struggles to comprehend strong experiences like the fighter who, having been knocked out, cannot remember the last few punches.

People only gradually "come to their senses" after a trauma like prematurity. During this time of waiting, you may relive what happened many times as you attempt to gain a better understanding, a better adjustment. However, this process is frustratingly slow because of ongoing concern for your child.

Coping with a baby in an intensive care unit makes it impossible to concentrate on working through your trauma, especially if your baby becomes worse or faces surgery. As you sit home depressed, confused, and lonely because your baby is not there, realize that this flood of uncomfortable emotions is a necessary part of the adjustment process. You will only frustrate yourself by expecting to put your fears behind you because, like an earthquake, prematurity has aftershocks. Your patience may temporarily desert you, but it will be the best friend you have.

The long wait has the benefit of allowing you to recover without the constant demands of a baby in the home, giving you needed time. Trips to the hospital and routine household chores are more than enough for someone who has been through what you have.

Like most premature parents waiting for their baby's homecoming, Lauren and I were on an emotional roller coaster. She became seriously depressed for an eternity of nine days. Even now, as psychologists, neither of us understand everything that happened. We hope that by describing common emotions many parents feel at this time you will be helped in understanding your own.

Post Partum Depression and Recovery

It is well-known that women who give birth to healthy, full-term babies often experience a period of depression (Brewer, 1978; Spock, 1976). Thus, if you become depressed, it is hardly surprising. Many premature mothers, in addition, feel responsible for the prematurity as if they alone had the power to control the length of pregnancy. Mothers often blame themselves for everything. Regrets about drinking, under or over exercising, insufficient resting, continuing intercourse, smoking, and traveling are common.

Something has gone wrong with your body. You need not atone for it. You have to take care of yourself, your family, and your baby. Being absorbed in guilt over an accident will make your task that much more, unnecessarily, difficult.

If I knew how to inoculate people against post partum depression, I'd be a happy psychologist. My bleakest moments occurred not when Christopher was born and in danger of death. I hit the bottom while Lauren was depressed, when our son was stabilizing and beginning to grow. My depression was caused by the inner acknowledgement that our ordeal was not over despite Christopher's becoming healthy. I believe that some guilt and depression are probably necessary for a long-term emotional recovery from prematurity. However, I wish that this were not the case because a serious depression is very unpleasant.

Maternal Depression, by Lauren Leslie-Hynan

The ideal image of motherhood contains a scene of parents beaming with joy as they hold their newborn baby in the mother's hospital room. The mother looks tired but happy after a relatively painless vaginal labor.

This is the image I carried with me throughout pregnancy. I looked forward to a "natural" childbirth as the most intimate experience between husband and wife. The power of this image became clearer to me when later contrasting it with my very different

64

experience of giving birth.

When I received general anesthesia, I was afraid
that I would never awaken and my baby would be
stillborn. Coming to in the recovery room, I felt as
if I'd been robbed--I had no baby beside me. I
thought, "Do I have to go through another pregnancy to
get my dream, my ideal, fulfilled?" Two nights later,
someone took a baby from me during a dream in which I
felt a sense of loss so deep it was almost a physical
pain.

The day after, my obstetrician asked if I were
distancing myself from the baby. Things had, in fact,
gotten to the point where I was not even able to look
at Christopher's picture. After my doctor left, a
wonderful, understanding nurse came in and asked if
I'd cried yet.

I'd always been able to cry easily before, but
this time I had held onto my tears, afraid to let go.
All I needed was permission and, gratefully, I sobbed
into the arms of two caring nurses, mourning for a
lost dream, for a loss of control over my life.
Prematurity had reminded me of how vulnerable I was, a
realization no one faces easily. For those of us who
want control, it's doubly hard.

I spent the first month after surgery gaining
strength, living with recurrent high blood pressure,
visiting Christopher, and coping with my emotions.
The first week home contained great highs and lows.
The first two days, despite my happiness at being
discharged, there was little I could do without
quickly tiring. I wanted to gain strength but didn't
know how.

I became hyper-vigilant about my body. Desiring
to lower my blood pressure, I was at once fearful of
overexertion while pushing myself to exercise. I was
also taking a type of hypertension medication which,
given in large dosages, causes fatigue and depression.

The fifth day home, which was quite beautiful, I
took a half-mile walk. But, returning home,
everything caught up with me. The intense fatigue was
so terrifying, I became afraid of falling asleep for
fear I would die. I asked Michael to reassure me I
wasn't going crazy and, somewhat comforted but not
totally believing him, relaxed enough to sleep.

Although that week was my lowest point, the next month was hardly smooth. I found I had few emotional resources and slowly learned to save myself for what was really important, as difficult as I found this. For example, one morning I made two short professional calls that exhausted me so totally I staggered to the couch and slept for two hours. From such experiences, I began to listen to my body and take one day at a time.

My calendar, which detailed this period, showed relapses following attempts to return to normal. My world narrowed to our home and the hospital. I spent most of each day in bed, preparing for the forty-five mile trip to the nursery. When just washing my hair left me too tired to visit Christopher, I was angry and guilty for having made my appearance a higher priority.

Whenever the hospital staff gave us new responsibilities, such as feeding or changing, I was drained. Yet each new duty meant Christopher was improving, and we were beginning to take over our roles as parents. The more contact we had, the stronger bonding became, and the more I missed him when I returned home.

I avoided interacting with anyone other than Michael, our son, and the hospital staff. It was as if everyone else were alien to me because they didn't understand what we were going through. To explain again and again was too much to bear. My friends found my withdrawal particularly hard because they wanted to help me.

I am a person who can usually ask for help, but this time I wanted only those people around me who intimately knew what was happening. I cried almost daily and remember saying I didn't want Christopher to be raised by a mother who cried all the time. But those tears were a part of a healing process.

Recovery finally got easier when I stopped fighting myself. Initially, I had thought that I should not have been so upset but, unable to snap out of the blues, I ended up feeling worse. I regained some control over my life by accepting my emotions; thus, I took the pressure off my recovery.

I slowly grew stronger, found that short periods
of energy and joy returned, and learned to trust
myself again. After Christopher came home, my healing
was sufficient to allow for fully involved parenting.
I came to believe I could be a good mother.

Paternal Depression

Many fathers have an ideal image of their family
as being secure, comfortable, and well provided for.
The arrival of a new baby is supposed to enhance the
family. But family stability disappears after a
premature birth.

A father may find himself in a situation wherein
he is the only family member living in the home. The
wife may be in one hospital, the baby in a second, and
the other children with relatives. His time may be
spent traveling between work, the hospitals, and an
empty house. When the wife and children do return
home, the baby may still be struggling for months
before discharge. Although parents may have
anticipated that a new infant would disrupt the family
a bit, one does not bargain for this.

A father's bewilderment and confusion stem from
many sources: frustration over not being able to help
the wife or baby, depression because the birth was not
normal, fear as the infant's recovery goes from up to
down, helplessness in the face of growing debt from
medical bills, and guilt over any number of things
that might have been better handled.

During the long weeks of confusion and waiting,
Lauren and I would look at each other and say, "All it
is, is hard. All this is, is hard." Just saying this
helped us realize that, even though these were very
difficult times, we could cope and not be crushed. It
also acknowledged that hard times were going to be
with us for yet awhile.

We had hope there was light at the end of the
tunnel, although the light seemed very faint, and
occasionally we could not see it. Our train to
recovery was moving very slowly. Any time we
anticipated a quick solution, we were disappointed.
We learned the true virtue of patience.

I was able to cope with Lauren's depression by
observing its cycles. While she periodically seemed

to be coming out of it, after a few hours of energy
and a bit of cheer, fatigue would return. If I
allowed my spirits to rise with hers, they would drop
with hers. I accepted the normal levels of
frustration and depression which this crisis entailed.
It was all I could do.

During this time, the family will generally look
to the father as a pillar of strength, and men may
have a tendency to give without asking in return.
Further, a husband's customary source of support, his
wife, may not be able to help. It is important not to
let pride get in the way of talking to and taking
comfort from one's friends and relatives.

However, don't think of your wife as an invalid.
Although she may not be able to offer the same degree
of support as is customary, she will feel better if
you both try to help each other. Giving, on whatever
level we are capable, makes us feel better about
ourselves.

Two months after Christopher came home, I was
still quite upset and depressed. I entered therapy,
gaining relief as the therapist helped me put my
feelings and Christopher's birth into perspective. If
you feel counseling is necessary, allow yourself to
get it as soon as possible; your depression will lift
that much sooner. Although many people only think of
seeing a therapist as a last resort, a terrible
admission that they cannot solve their own problems,
this is nonsense. Entering therapy is a wise
acknowledgement of a time of stress and crisis.

Also remember your friends are your friends
because you share confidences. If you need emotional
support and do not ask for it, you can expect some of
your friends to be angry. (A few of mine were.) They
want to help, and you minimize your friendship by not
letting them.

There is another stress which is felt strongly by
many fathers. This is the financial cost of
prematurity. Lauren and I were quite fortunate in
that insurance paid for almost all of our hospital
bills. Some of you may find that your insurance
covers very little of the medical costs. It is not
unusual to be shocked by a hospital bill of over
$100,000. Dreams of a home, car, or college for your
children will be shattered.

I worried a lot about money when I didn't know
how much the insurance would pay. I stopped worrying
when I saw I had no control over the matter. We would
never have stopped Christopher's medical treatments
just because they were putting us into debt. I knew I
would live with whatever happened.

Be aware that the cost of hospital trips can be
listed as a medical deduction on your income taxes.
Lauren and I deducted the 2,800 miles we drove. Many
of you will have greater travel expenses than this.
Be sure to keep a record of hospital visits and
mileage driven. Also remember to add charges for
parking and tolls.

The Need to Communicate

There are times when the emotions you are
experiencing will match your spouse's. But when your
emotions do not match--for instance, when one of you
is angry and the other is sad--this may be a cause for
misunderstanding and disharmony. For this reason,
many parents have stressed the necessity of continued
communication (Nance, 1982). Communication will lead
to better understanding, which will bring more
patience and love.

Many parents report that prematurity strengthened
their marriage. A crisis often brings people closer
together, uniting them against danger. But when the
Alarm Stage is over and both spouses are in the
Resistance Stage, there is a greater chance of marital
conflict. The entire family is getting less emotional
comfort. It is, therefore, essential to express your
feelings, hopes, fears, needs, and desires. You will
not always attain satisfaction, but you will know
more, and there will be no worries about what the
other person is thinking.

The importance of communication extends to all
family members. Having a premature sibling places
extra stress on children. Most children expect some
changes in the family when a new baby is born, even
though they may not anticipate what those changes will
be. This expectation may cause them insecurity when
they realize you are upset. They may also be
disappointed because you haven't brought the baby home
with you. Because it is difficult for children to
cope with confused feelings, you must encourage them
to confide in you.

Children sometimes incorrectly blame themselves for bad things. When your children notice you are distraught, they may think they have done something wrong. In addition, some children blame themselves for prematurity if they previously did not want another brother or sister. They may need your reassurance.

Many parents have questions about how much to tell their children about the baby's condition. Since children's fear of the unknown is usually worse than their fear of hospitals or sickness, I encourage you to bring your children to visit their sibling (if hospital rules permit). You should prepare them by showing pictures of the infant and explaining the equipment used in the intensive care unit. When they understand that ventilators and IVs are there to help the baby breathe and eat, they will be much less afraid.

Remember your children may lose interest in the visit before you do. One parent or a friend can take them on a walk if they become bored to extend the visit peaceably.

When you return home, give your children time to express their feelings about the visit. If they are unable to talk about this, have them draw a picture of their sibling. You can also play a game of hospital and pretend to take care of your baby.

Some parents have found a special book, The Frogs Have a Baby, a Very Small Baby, by Jerri Oehler (unpublished manuscript) to be useful in explaining prematurity to children. It is a cartoon coloring book of a frog family with a premature baby frog. The mommy and daddy frogs explain why the baby must stay in the hospital. There are also pictures of hospital equipment and frog doctors and nurses. This book can be adapted to fit your family situation.

The need to communicate also applies to friends and relatives. You will find that almost everyone is as ignorant of prematurity as you were before your baby was born. Since friends and relatives may not know how to help you, it is up to you to communicate your needs straightforwardly. Your parents can be both especially helpful when they understand these needs and especially stressful when they do not understand. They may intrude in your lives in undesired ways, or avoid you and their grandchildren out of fear. It is only through open communication that you can understand and support each other.

Sometimes communication can result in temporary difficulties. Someone, with the best of intentions, may try to help and end up intruding. Honest feedback may result in hurt. But the long-term benefits of communicating are much greater than the short-term risk of offense.

In my case, my mother wanted to live with me while Lauren was hospitalized so she could take care of cooking and cleaning while offering me support. However, at the time, I wanted to be alone. I was so busy between visits to Lauren and Christopher and teaching at the university that home was my only refuge. I know I hurt my mother when I asked her not to come, but this hurt was healed when she realized I still needed her support through telephone conversations and visits to Christopher.

Another example occurred during Lauren's depression. After returning home, she received a long distance call from a very close friend and, sobbing, felt obligated to tell the whole story. After only a minute I could tell she was draining herself, so I took the phone and explained to the friend we would return the call when able. Although I was abrupt, the friend understood. We later received a beautiful card, letting us know that she and her husband would even fly in to stay with us. It was exactly the kind of emotional support we needed.

You will find that, even though you communicate your needs, some people will not be able to empathize with you. Because of this, many parents have found that their only source of comfort came from talking with other parents of premature infants. Frequently, communities will have support groups started by parents of premature infants. The hospital staff should know if one exists in your area. I strongly suggest that you call one of the members and go to the meetings. You will find much comfort in talking to those who have been through the crises you are experiencing (Minde, Schosenberg, & Morton, 1980).

If you have problems finding a local group, you can contact a new international organization, Parent Care - Parents of Premature and High-Risk Infants,

International. The address of Parent Care is:
University of Utah Medical Center, 50 North Medical
Drive, Room 2A210, Salt Lake City, Utah, 84132.
Parent Care has information on parent groups
throughout the world. You can join Parent Care or,
for a nominal charge, you can receive their newsletter
and a resource directory containing current
information about parenting high-risk infants.

If there are no support groups in your area, ask
your neonatologist if he or she would recommend other
premature parents you could talk with. Try to find
parents whose baby is between one and two years old.
In this stage of the crisis, the experience is still
fresh in their minds. They can assure you by example
that, even though your lives are difficult now, things
will get better.

The crises of premature birth take their toll
over time. The disruptions of family stability exact
a high cost in emotional turmoil. At times, the
continued struggle may seem to be too much. Indeed,
many parents have told me that they found themselves
wishing their baby had died, so they would not have to
endure the continued pain of prematurity.

These parents felt that they were terrible for
having such feelings, and many were reluctant to share
their dark secrets. But even these feelings are
normal reactions to prematurity. I encourage you to
communicate with those people who can empathize with
you. You will find out that you are not alone, and
this support can help you through your difficult
times.

Relating to the Intensive Care Staff

As you make more visits to see your baby, you
will get to know many of the people who work in the
neonatal intensive care unit. The various staff
members have different types of training, experience,
and responsibilities.

The neonatologist has the ultimate responsibility
for your infant. You may also meet neonatology
fellows and pediatric residents. The fellows have
completed at least three years training in pediatrics
and are studying for advanced licensing in
neonatology. The residents are generally young
doctors who are completing their training to be

certified as pediatricians. Some, even all, of these
doctors may change during your baby's hospitalization
when the usual rotations occur.

You will have the closest contact with the
nurses. Neonatal nurses are registered nurses who
often have special training in pediatrics. It is
likely one of the neonatal nurses will be assigned to
your baby as a primary care nurse. When this nurse
is off shift, other nurses may have primary care of
the infant. The nursing staff is less likely to
change during your baby's stay.

The staff of any neonatal intensive care unit is
highly trained and dedicated. They have chosen to
work in an area where crises are frequent, and they
are very competent in what they do. The relationships
you develop with the doctors and nurses become very
important. You are trusting your baby to their care,
and very often you will find their skills bring you
comfort and security.

However, at times, parents may feel jealousy and
anger toward the medical staff, reactions to the
stress and frustration of prematurity. Because
parents are usually only able to visit the nursery for
a few hours each day, they are aware that their baby
has constant attention from the nurses. Parents may
wonder if their baby knows who its real parents are
and if their baby will form an attachment to the
nurses in their stead.

But there is little or no basis for this fear.
It is the quality of parental contact that matters,
not the quantity. During the time Christopher was
hospitalized, he was with Lauren and myself for an
average of one-and-a-half hours per day over forty-one
days. He, obviously, had much more contact with the
medical staff, yet Christopher developed a beautiful,
loving attachment to us.

You may also become angry at times with the
staff. If you are frustrated with the ups and downs
of your baby's recovery, you may second-guess the
doctors. A nurse may give you inaccurate or
incomplete information; a doctor may make a comment
that terrifies you until you later discover there was
nothing to worry about. You may fly off the handle,
but the staff has had years of experience with
premature parents, and they know that it is normal, in

your situation, to get upset (Kemp & Page, 1986). If your anger is justified, they will listen closely to what you say. If it is not, a simple apology should reestablish your relationship on a good level.

When Lauren and I got angry, we avoided the medical staff but, after realizing this was foolish, we began interacting again. By doing so, we were able to regain the confidence in Christopher's care that was so important to us. In times of conflict, it will help to remember that the staff is also under a great deal of stress coping with their own reactions to the life-and-death struggles of many babies (Marshall & Kasman, 1982). A common appreciation of the stresses on both sides can go a long way toward restoring communication.

In some hospitals you can read your baby's medical charts. If you are curious about your baby's charts, there are two things you should do. First, you should find out the hospital's policy. Second, if you are allowed to read the charts, you should ask yourself a question: "Am I the kind of person who will benefit from reading the information (often very technical) and knowing everything? Or, will the information just upset and confuse me?"

The charts are written for the medical staff, not the parents. Often facts are written in medical abbreviations without elaborations. Special tests will be ordered and their results will be unintelligible to you. On the average, the charts give more questions to parents than answers. They can cause anxiety.

If you feel sure that the medical staff will tell you of any major problems, and if you only care about things like weight gain and whether your baby had a peaceful night, then I suggest that you don't read the charts. You can ask your baby's nurse or doctor the questions you wish. They can then read the charts and give you the answers. On the other hand, if you need to know everything (like Lauren and I did), go ahead and read the charts. If you don't understand something, or an entry makes you upset, please ask your nurse or doctor about it. You don't want to find yourselves worrying about something for a few days, and then find out that it meant nothing when you finally ask about it.

<u>Realizing</u> <u>Your</u> <u>Baby</u> <u>Will</u> <u>Live</u>

The time of your baby's hospitalization is a slow process of adaptation and, although the chances are great your baby will come home as healthy as any full-term child, there are many hills and valleys in between. You will be changing your perceptions about your baby's health constantly.

Believing your baby will live a healthy life depends upon positive signs from treatment. When your baby no longer needs a ventilator or oxygen hood, you have some indication that the struggle for survival is being won. When intravenous feeding is no longer necessary and your baby is breathing room air, your confidence increases. Finally, your baby no longer requires an isolette. As you watch your baby gain weight, you begin to believe that the worst is over.

But it takes time for parents to have realistic feelings about premature babies. Christopher was home for a few months before we finally began to accept him as a normal baby and not a baby in danger. In this regard, we were like many parents (Danko, Nagy, & Holmes, 1982). As time goes by, and as you know your baby better, you will find the appropriate level of concern.

At some point you will realize that your baby could come home in two or three weeks. This is the time for discharge planning. The hospital staff will assist you in getting ready for your baby's homecoming. There are many things to learn.

Make sure that you know how to diaper and bathe your baby. Get information on where to obtain clothing, premie diapers, and a crib. Some parents will need special instruction on their baby's diet and any medications their baby may need. Other parents may need to arrange for visits by home care nurses, especially if their baby comes home requiring special equipment like an apnea monitor or ventilator. These parents will also need to be trained in how to use the equipment.

When the time comes to arrange your child's discharge date, you will feel rushed, even though the hospitalization has lasted a psychological eternity. Because Christopher gained two ounces a day during his last two weeks in the nursery, his release came more rapidly than expected. We had to do many things seemingly at once: learn to bathe him, paint his nursery, set up the crib and changing table, buy clothes.... We didn't have time to buy enough bottles until after he was home!

And then the day comes. You will walk out of the hospital with your baby in your arms and you will go <u>home</u>. Regardless of whether he has been hospitalized for one week, two months, or a year, you will feel a great sense of thankfulness. You will be nervous but very, very proud. Swelling in your breasts will be a magnificent feeling of having done it. Your baby has proven a strong fighter; you have struggled more than you ever thought you could; your family has endured.

At last, your baby can smell fresh air and feel the sun upon its face.

I hope you savor that moment. It is a reward you truly deserve.

Chapter Five - References

Brewer, G. (1978). Cooperative childbirth: The woman-centered approach. In G. Brewer (Ed.), The Pregnancy After Thirty Workbook (pp. 79-132). Emmanus, PA: Rodale Press.

Danko, M., Nagy, J., & Holmes, D. (1982). The effects of prematurity and illness on parents' perceptions of their infants. Paper presented at the meeting of the Midwestern Psychological Association, Minneapolis.

Kemp, V. & Page, C. (1986). The psychosocial impact of a high-risk pregnancy on the family. Journal of Obstetric, Gynecologic, and Neonatal Nursing, 15, 232-236.

Marshall, R. & Kasman, C. (1982). Burnout. In R. Marshall, C. Kasman, & L. Cape (Eds.), Coping with Caring for Sick Newborns (pp. 5-15). Philadelphia: W. B. Saunders.

Minde, K., Schosenberg, N., & Morton, P. (1980). Self help groups in a premature nursery - A controlled evaluation. Journal of Pediatrics, 96 (5), 933-940.

Nance, S. (1982). Premature Babies: A Handbook for Parents. New York: Arbor House.

Oehler, J. (unpublished manuscript). The Frogs Have a Baby, A Very Small Baby. Available for $1.50 from Jerri Oehler, R.N., 210 Landsbury Drive, Durham, NC 27707.

Spock, B. (1976). Infant and Child Care. New York: Pocket Books.

CHAPTER SIX

YOUR BABY IS HOME

Learning to live with your premature baby twenty-four hours a day brings the next phase of adjustment. You need to learn how to structure your lives to find what is best for you, your other children, and your infant. Many parents experience homecoming as joyful, but this honeymoon will last only a few days or weeks. Although you will find a renewed energy and sense of excitement in what you do, the excitement soon fades as the task of having a newborn at home becomes hard work. This work is often harder for premature than for full-term parents due to the general phenomenon of parental over-concern.

Parental Over-concern

Many parents show more concern for their baby than necessary. They may check diapers constantly, watch over sleep to check their baby's breathing, or lie awake listening for little cries of distress. Premature parents are more likely to show excessive over-concern for fear that the baby may, once again, edge close to death. However, the great majority of you have little reason to worry. Although some infants do come home with continued apnea or require ventilator care and, thus, demand constant vigilance, most are quite healthy.

Lauren and I incessantly monitored Christopher upon his homecoming because of our continued perception of him as sick, despite his being fine. It was difficult to stop thinking of our son as special, but it was necessary. Such worrying on our part was exhausting.

If you have questions about how closely to watch your baby, ask the neonatologist. Unless given special precautions, you can begin to accept your infant as normal.

Because it is important to guard against exhaustion, I suggest the following:

1. Unless circumstances force you to do so, do not sleep in the same room with your baby. You will hear cries even if your baby is two

or three rooms away. You do not need to be awakened by a baby's normal movements.

2. Have a good friend or one of the baby's grandparents spend a few weeks living with you to help in caring for the infant and your home.

3. Fathers should help out by being home more often and assisting with feedings and household chores.

4. Limit the number of visits to your home by friends and relatives since these can prove tiring.

5. Unless you have a specific reason for doing so, do not weigh your infant daily as readings can be misleading due to normal elimination. Either weigh once a week (at most) or wait until you visit the pediatrician.

6. Since your baby will probably come home on three-hour feedings which give you little rest, consider adopting a schedule of family responsibilities for cooking, feeding, cleaning, and other chores.

When Christopher was on a three-hour schedule, he was hungry during the night at approximately 10:00 p.m., 1:00 a.m., and 4:00 a.m. Lauren and I decided she would breast-feed at 10:00 p.m. and 1:00 a.m., while I would bottle-feed at 4:00 a.m. This allowed each of us to have a six- to seven-hour period in which to sleep.

Remember, feedings may be given in the baby's room by only one of you, allowing the other to rest. The schedule that works is the one of maximum benefit to all concerned.

For Parents of Premature Twins

Parents of multiple premature infants have special difficulties. Not only do they have more than one sick baby, one of these babies is usually sicker than the other(s). Thus, emotional adjustment becomes more complex.

Many parents of premature twins report they have initially been more concerned with the sicker baby and then felt guilty over neglecting the healthier one. The situation is exacerbated when one baby has been discharged while the other remains hospitalized. Unfortunately, in this dilemma, all the possible solutions are less than desirable.

One frequent coping scheme is to have each parent primarily caring for one of the twins. Although this works practically, it hinders equal bonding with the babies. Things are further complicated by a tendency for both parents to bond to one twin over the other. (Some parents attach themselves more to the sicker baby while others grow closer to the infant they believe has the best chance to live.)

The goal of loving both babies equally is impossible to attain during the early stages of the prematurity crisis. Thus, premature parents of twins may have a slower rate of adjustment.

Parents of premature twins have also told me of another unique problem which occurred when one of their babies died while the sibling survived healthily. After grieving about the death, the parents focused their attentions and hopes on the healthier infant. Over time, this child became stronger, and the parents accepted that it would live. However, the parents became unexpectedly saddened again for the baby who had died. (Anniversaries such as birthdays are especially difficult times.) These parents realized that having twins had prevented them from mourning as much as they could have and that they had to re-experience grief as part of their adjustment process.

If your twins survive and grow, you will feel twice blessed in addition to knowing firsthand that raising them is more than twice as hard as raising one child. It is all right if you love one of your babies more than the other. It is also all right if you feel grief years after one of them has died. These are feelings that go with the territory.

The Stages of Parental Adjustment

After you have been home a few weeks, it will help you to look back and appreciate what you have been through. Four stages of parental adjustment to

prematurity were described in 1965 by Drs. Gerald
Caplan, Edward Mason, and David Kaplan, neonatology
experts. Looking back at how you survived the first
three stages makes it easier to resolve your last
stage.

The first stage occurred after your baby was
born. Then you prepared yourselves for the
possibility that your baby might die. You hoped with
all your might that your baby would live, but
anticipatory grief insulated you from the deep pain of
possible death.

The second stage involved the mother's adjustment
to guilt. You mothers faced the fact that you did not
have a normal labor and delivery. You wondered what
went wrong and blamed yourselves for many things (both
reasonable and unreasonable). After accepting the
failure to deliver normally, you parents moved to the
third stage.

The third stage was the resumption of relating to
your baby. As your baby stabilized, gained weight,
and became more active you began the process of
bonding. You slowly gave up anticipatory grief and
began to relate to your baby as someone who would be
with your family forever.

Your last stage began with understanding the
special needs of your premature baby. It involved
learning how to hold, feed, diaper, and bathe someone
so tiny. During the early part of stage four you
recognized that your baby was an infant with special
needs. These needs then became your major concerns.
When you think of the effort you put into adjusting to
these stages, you will realize that you have been
through a lot.

As you look back, you may wonder how you made it
this far. Yet, realizing that the worst is over is a
sign that you are approaching the end of the last
stage. You have one more task remaining before you
can become just regular parents.

There comes a time in the fourth stage when you
need to integrate your baby into your family. How
quickly you do this will depend upon how you feel
about the health of your baby.

As parents watch their baby become healthy and grow, their consideration of their baby changes. This change in concept is important for two reasons. One reason is for your psychological well being. When you begin to regard your baby as normal, you can breathe a sigh of relief. If there are no special precautions, your fears and anxieties can be reduced. You can go from the Resistance stage of fighting stress back to your normal patterns of living.

The second reason for the change in concept is the psychological development of your baby. Most people believe that a child's self-concept is greatly influenced by the child's relationship with its parents. If the parents believe that their baby is unusual, it is likely that the baby will grow up feeling different. But if the parents treat their baby as normal, the baby will grow up with the self-concept of being normal and healthy.

This transition in the way you think of your baby generally comes slowly. You will often think of your experience. People who watch your baby grow will remark, "You would never know that she (or he) was premature." But these reminders will come less and less often. As this happens, I hope that you will begin to think of your baby as a normal baby and treat your baby as a healthy baby.

Unfortunately, 20% to 30% of babies weighing less than 1500 grams at birth will have significant physical problems throughout their lives (Cohen et al., 1982; Ment, Scott, Ehrenkranz, Rothman, Duncan, & Warshaw, 1982). So some parents will always regard their baby as special due to physical handicaps. However, it is important to treat your child as no more special than he or she actually is. If your child is handicapped, you will always feel some sadness. But once you have accepted your child, your lives will be as enriched as those of the parents of any child.

Your Baby's Future Medical Treatment

After your baby has been discharged, you will be concerned with future medical checkups. You may bring your baby back to a follow-up clinic at the hospital where the intensive care unit was or go to a pediatrician who is not a neonatologist. Some parents will do both.

It is important to find a pediatrician with whom you have a good working relationship. If you already have children and trust their doctor, you may have no extra work. However, because many of you will be first-time parents, you may ask for referrals from the hospital neonatologist.

Regardless of how you find your pediatrician, it is crucial that you trust him or her with your infant. Lauren and I went along for our son's first office examination and were surprised to find that our pediatrician regarded Christopher as a normal, average baby. He, in fact, asked no special questions about the prematurity. We were assured that we could call to ask questions or bring Christopher in whenever we felt something was wrong. When we have called, he has always called us back within an hour. Although our son does not get sick more often than any other average child, we still worry. Having a pediatrician in whom we have faith has helped us immensely.

Because this faith is so important, be careful in chosing your pediatrician. Many neonatologists believe that premature infants should continue to have follow-up care done by neonatologists. So ask the advice of the neonatologist who knows your child the best. Confidence in your baby's future medical care will be a source of comfort to you.

The Stress of a New Baby

Having a newborn in the home is a twenty-four hour job. A baby disrupts one's lifestyle and family pattern. Whenever a baby needs something, parents generally stop what they are doing and tend to the baby. Even when they try to ignore cries, they are distracted.

A baby will keep you from enjoying some of your previous comforts. Things like a quiet, uninterrupted dinner, a full night's sleep, or thirty minutes of free time will disappear.

A newborn in the house gets all the attention. Psychologists have used the term "sibling rivalry" to describe the negative reaction in children when they have a new brother or sister come home. Instead of "sibling rivalry," I like the term "family rivalry" because it includes the entire family.

When a baby comes home, all family members receive less comfort, attention, and emotional support than they are used to. This becomes irritating at times. Older children may regress to gain attention, fathers may not be able to unwind with the evening paper because of additional household duties, and mothers may feel they are getting less comfort from husbands and children while the baby occupies everyone's time. In family rivalry, everyone is jealous, not only of the baby, but of any family member who is stealing attention.

Although family rivalry has no specific cure, its alleviation comes from the open expression of needs, frustrations, and concerns. It is always difficult, if not impossible, to read each other's minds. If you expect that your spouse and children will automatically and intuitively understand you, you will be frequently disappointed. Everyone in your family may feel they are giving far and away more than they are receiving. Talking about resentment eases tension, and workable compromises can be explored.

You can cuddle with your spouse while the baby sleeps, have your other children feed the infant and fold diapers, and spend quality time with your children that does not involve the baby. Everyone needs to give a little more when family rivalry causes problems.

At different times during the first few months, many parents secretly wish they never had a baby and would like to dispose of the infant with the bath water. A friend of ours has said, "Just when you feel like throwing your baby off the treetops, she smiles." After the initial honeymoon period, the rewards can seem few. But, during the precious moments when your baby smiles, lifts its head, and sits up; it will all feel very worthwhile.

Any newborn, but especially a premature newborn, will put stress on your sexual relationship (Fischman, Rankin, Soeken, & Lenz, 1986). One reason for this is simple fatigue. Many parents are tired all the time during the first few months. When the baby is asleep and there is no housework or childcare to do, the first thing you may desire is sleep. Even if you do find some free time and you are not tired, you may wish to cherish it by yourself with no demands. Fatigue can also cause you to lose interest in sex or to be out of sexual synchrony with your spouse's moods.

Another stress upon sexuality is fear of having another pregnancy. After having had one premature child, any subsequent pregnancy becomes high-risk. The odds of any woman having a premature baby are about twelve to one. After having had one premature birth, the odds increase to approximately four to one (Henig & Fletcher, 1983; Nance, 1982). Fear of repeating the prematurity experience can put a stop to much of the spontaneity and joy in any sexual relationship.

Further, both spouses may be preoccupied with the anxiety, guilt, and frustration that accompany prematurity. You may feel it is not right to enjoy yourselves while your baby is in danger.

An added stress to your sexuality is the expectation that your sex lives should return to normal quickly. But if you press for romance you are sure to be disappointed and frustrated because many things will interfere.

If the mother has had surgery, her scars may make her feel less feminine. If parents are always vigilant about apnea monitors, they will not be paying attention to the joys in their bodies. Nursing mothers may not want to become aroused because they fear they will lose milk. This can frustrate fathers who may already be trying to adjust to a lover who is less shapely than before. These are sensitive subjects which are bound to inhibit sex. Not talking about your feelings can only make things worse.

I have talked with parents whose sex lives have been disrupted for two or three years following a high-risk birth. Often it is just as difficult to re-learn the joys of sex as it was to learn them in the first place. Pressures for sex and a quick return to romance will just make things worse. (Some parents have helped themselves by agreeing to abstain from having sex or even planning it.) By taking the pressures off, parents can give themselves time to re-discover their feelings for each other.

As the pressures and stresses go away over time, you will find that your interest in and zeal for sex will grow stronger. As our interest in sex returned,

Lauren and I had the wonderful realization of, "Oh, yes, I remember now what it was like!" You need only be patient and strive to keep communicating for this to happen to you.

The fear of another prematurity will not go away easily, however. Some parents decide that they will never risk another pregnancy. For these parents a tubal ligation or vasectomy may be necessary before they can enjoy sex fully. Others decide to conceive again. Lauren and I, like most parents, are unsure. We have decided not to have another child in the near future, but have left open the possibility for later on. The choice is both very difficult and very personal.

If you do decide to have another child, it would be wise to prepare for the possibility of another premature birth. If your obstetrician is not a specialist in high-risk pregnancies, he or she may refer you to someone who is. Or you may decide to change to an high-risk obstetrician or a perinatologist affiliated with a hospital that has good neonatal facilities. When you are advised of the procedures available for managing high-risk pregnancies, you will have the best chance for a normal, full-term birth.

The Exhaustion Stage

I have written this book so that premature parents need never reach the Exhaustion Stage described by Selye (1956). Unfortunately, some parents do become physically and emotionally exhausted. If this happens, there are special things you can do.

You are exhausted when you have lost all ability to cope with even minor aspects of your life and, at such time, require help. It is essential that someone take care of you until you recover.

Sometimes exhausted individuals require hospitalization and benefit greatly from sessions with a psychotherapist. Other exhausted people need to escape home and family, taking a vacation with a friend or relative along who can provide them with care. (The spouse may provide the care if not too busy with the baby and family.)

87

In any case, exhaustion means you must, for your own good, make yourself your most important concern. It will very likely mean a separation from the infant.

Exhaustion can be defined as reaching the bottom of the pit. Most premature parents feel close to the bottom during their ordeal but rarely crash. It is important that you do whatever you can to avoid exhaustion.

If you do become exhausted, however, it is not cause for blame or shame. While feeling you have gone crazy, you have simply fallen victim to stress. When that stress has been removed you will recover, somewhat wiser and certainly older.

There is a tendency for people who have become exhausted to feel as though they have failed. Frequently, they lose self-esteem and fear others will regard them as less worthwhile. But exhaustion only indicates that one has succumbed to enormous pressure, nothing more. One's task is simply to recover and return to home and family.

Exhaustion occurs most often when people try to cope with prematurity by themselves. Communicating your feelings and asking for help are the best ways to avoid exhaustion.

Resolution of the Crises

Life becomes easier as your baby grows and develops. Over the months, you will stop listening for faint noises in the night. As your baby sleeps longer, so will you. When your baby turns over by itself and learns to crawl, you will have evidence of good development.

However, some premature parents worry excessively about development, about whether their baby is developmentally lagging. Lauren and I knew that Christopher crawled and walked later than expected, and he is also less coordinated than other children his age. But this delay has not been very important to us. As long as we see some development, even if slow, we are happy for we have a son we expect to see alive the next day.

Many parents come to recognize that they worry only when they continuously compare their baby with the developmental charts. When this gets too frustrating, some parents toss the charts away. It is more meaningful to compare your baby's development only to your baby.

When your baby learns to walk, negotiate stairs, and eat without much help, you will have more time to yourselves. Someday you will find yourselves sitting somewhere, perhaps looking at your baby. One of you (or both) will realize that the crisis is over. Indeed, when this happens you will also know that the crisis has been over for quite some time. You are the normal parents of a loved baby. You have endured and survived. You can be very proud of what you have done.

Even though the crisis has been resolved, the experiences of being a premature parent still remain. At the end of the crisis most parents realize that there is a positive side to having a premature baby. Yes, a positive side. If you are reading this before the resolution of your crisis you may (like Lauren) find it hard to believe that anything good could come from prematurity. But good does come.

There are very special moments that only premature parents can have. Many parents made promises to God, some to themselves, during the early stages of the crisis: "I'll be delighted, God, to wake up six times a night to a screaming, colicky baby, if only You will please let him live;" or "I'll be the kindest, most loving, and patient parent, I'll change my life and do things I never thought I could, if only my baby lives." These promises, which tend to be forgotten when the child grows up, deserve to be remembered.

When Christopher has been a monster all day, and I'm at the end of my rope, I sometimes recall the first few days of his life and my promises. My patience and love return immediately when I realize I have all I've asked for.

As premature parents you have been part of a life-and-death struggle. When you have seen life win, and when you are one of the reasons that your baby is alive, there is a special satisfaction that cannot be matched.

89

There is a place in the hearts of parents where only premature babies can go.

Chapter Six - References

Caplan, G., Mason, E., & Kaplan, D. (1965). Four studies of crisis in parents of prematures. Community Mental Health Journal, 1, 149-161.

Cohen, R., Stevenson, D., Malachowski, N., Ariagno, R., Kimble, K., Hopper, A., Johnson, J., Ueland, K., & Sunshine, P. (1982). Favorable results of neonatal intensive care for very low birth-weight infants. Pediatrics, 69, 621-625.

Fischman, S., Rankin, E., Soeken, K., & Lenz, E. (1986). Changes in sexual relationships in postpartum couples. Journal of Obstetric, Gynecologic, and Neonatal Nursing, 15, 58-63.

Henig, R., & Fletcher, B. (1983). Your Premature Baby. New York: Rawson Associates.

Ment, L., Scott, D., Ehrenkranz, R., Rothman, S., Duncan, C., & Warshaw, J. (1982). Neonates of greater than or equal to 1,250 grams birth weight: Prospective neurodevelopment evaluation during the first year postterm. Pediatrics, 70, 292-296.

Nance, S. (1982). Premature Babies: A Handbook for Parents. New York: Arbor House.

Selye, H. (1956). The Stress of Life. New York: McGraw-Hill.

ABOUT THE AUTHORS

Dr. Michael Hynan was born and raised in Chicago, IL. He attended St. Mary of the Lake Seminary in Niles, IL, and received his B.A. from the University of Notre Dame (1969). He received his M.S. (1971) and Ph.D. (1974) in Clinical Psychology from the University of Iowa. Dr. Hynan also completed an internship in the Division of Psychology, Department of Psychiatry at Ohio State University Hospitals. Since 1975 he has been a faculty member in the Psychology Department of the University of Wisconsin-Milwaukee, Milwaukee, WI, 53201 where he is currently an associate professor. Dr. Hynan has also been a visiting exchange professor in the Psychology Department at Justus-Liebig University in Giessen, West Germany. Dr. Hynan does research on aggressive behavior, personality, and psychotherapy. He also teaches courses in personality, abnormal behavior, and psychotherapy. He is a licensed clinical psychologist in the state of Wisconsin.

Dr. Lauren Leslie-Hynan was born in Haverhill, MA. She received her B.A. (1969) degree from the University of South Florida. She also received her M.A. (1972) in Child Development and her Ph.D. (1973) in Educational Psychology from the University of Iowa. Since 1974 she has been a faculty member at Marquette University, Milwaukee, WI where she is currently an associate professor. Dr. Leslie-Hynan does research on reading processes and reading disability. She also teaches courses in reading and educational psychology.